THINK FIRST

The Guilford School Practitioner Series

EDITORS

STEPHEN N. ELLIOTT, PhD
Vanderbilt University

JOSEPH C. WITT, PhD
Louisiana State University, Baton Rouge

Recent Volumes

Think First

ADDRESSING AGGRESSIVE BEHAVIOR
IN SECONDARY SCHOOLS

◆ ◆ ◆

Jim Larson

◆

THE GUILFORD PRESS
New York　　London

© 2005 The Guilford Press
A Division of Guilford Publications, Inc.
72 Spring Street, New York, NY 10012
www.guilford.com

Printed in the United States of America

This book is printed on acid-free paper.   #56526431

Last digit is print numbers: 9   8   7   6   5   4   3   2   1

Library of Congress Cataloging-in-Publication Data

Larson, Jim, 1942–
    Think first: addressing aggressive behavior in secondary schools / Jim Larson.
        p. cm. — (The Guilford school practitioner series)
    Includes bibliographical references and index.
    ISBN 1-59385-126-X (pbk.)
    1. Problem youth—Behavior modification—United States.   2. School violence—United States—Prevention.   3. High school students—United States—Psychology.   4. Middle school students—United States—Psychology.   I. Title   II. Series.
    LB 1060.2.L37 2005
    371.94—dc22
                                                                    2004021332

About the Author

◆

Jim Larson, PhD, is Professor of Psychology and Director of the School Psychology Program at the University of Wisconsin–Whitewater. He is also a member of the Scientific Board of the Melissa Institute for Violence Prevention and Treatment of Victims of Violence. Before moving to the University of Wisconsin–Whitewater, Dr. Larson was a school psychologist with the Milwaukee Public Schools in Milwaukee, Wisconsin, and the lead psychologist with the Milwaukee schools' Violence Prevention Program. His principal research interests include the treatment of aggression in children and adolescents, school violence prevention, and training procedures in school psychology. He is coauthor (with John E. Lochman) of *Helping School-children Cope with Anger: A Cognitive-Behavioral Intervention*, published by The Guilford Press.

Preface

◆

Interpersonal aggression among students is an unfortunate fact of life in America's middle and high schools. According to the National Center for Educational Statistics, in the year 2001, 33% of students in grades 9 through 12 reported that they had been in physical fights in the previous 12 months, and 13% reported that they had fought on school property. Although male students were more likely to have been in fights, 24% of female students reported that they had been in physical fights in the previous year and that 7% of this fighting took place on school property (DeVoe et al., 2002). In the current era of standards-based education and federal mandates that require schools to ensure a safe learning environment for all students, schools are under increasing pressure to address this problem effectively.

Fighting and other forms of physical aggression in the secondary school setting arise from a complex interaction of numerous intrapersonal and environmental factors. A diverse assemblage of middle and high school adolescents is brought together in an often crowded, closed space for 7 hours per day, 5 days per week, and this makes the likelihood of aggressive confrontations almost inevitable. Individual student risk factors such as poor anger management skills, emotional–behavioral disabilities, impulsivity, academic disengagement, and favorable dispositions for aggression serve only to increase the potential volatility. In addition, in many communities students come to school from home and street environments in which aggression may be an adaptive survival necessity, trained and reinforced from early in life. In response, secondary-level administrators, teachers, and supportive services personnel struggle, often heroically, to provide discipline structures, counseling, and diverse educational opportunities to help create safe and orderly learning environments for all students. This book is designed to assist them in this critically important task.

In the 1970s and 1980s, I was a school psychologist in a major urban school district. During that time, I served two high schools and a large middle school, all located in the central city. The late 1980s were difficult years for urban adolescents. Jobs were leaving the city and gangs and drugs were moving in. As Walinsky (1995) wrote:

> What we experienced from 1985 on was a conjunction of two terrible arrivals. One train carried the legacy of the 1970s, the children of the explosion of illegitimacy and parental abandonment. Crack arrived on the same timetable and unloaded at the same station. (p. 52)

Juvenile street crime was soaring to record levels, and schools were the recipients of its overflow. In 1988, stung by sensational media coverage of a number of violent incidents in the secondary schools, the school system funded an initiative that was identified as the "Violence Reduction Program." In spite of its imposing title, the new program was in reality only the reallocation of two individuals—a fellow school psychologist and me—to full-time involvement in the problem. In 1988, school violence was beginning to be taken seriously, but certainly not seriously enough. It would need to spread to the suburbs for that to eventually happen.

The 2 years I spent talking to administrators, researching strategies, running anger management groups, and conducting countless staff development workshops for the Violence Reduction Program convinced me that even in the most difficult of circumstances, motivated people with the right tools can do extraordinary things for high-risk students. Administrators who recognized that excessive exclusionary discipline was exacerbating the problem and incorporated more skills-based consequences began to make a difference. Teachers who diversified instruction and enhanced their classroom management abilities increased student academic engagement and lessened the need for disciplinary office referrals. School psychologists and guidance counselors who replaced their ineffective therapy procedures with focused, research-supported interventions began to see positive outcomes.

The world of the secondary school student has changed in many ways in the past 15 years, but the negative effects of poverty, drugs, overcrowding, aged facilities, and weakened family influence still hold considerable sway. Although these problems continue to present challenges, recent years have seen an impressive growth in research designed to address them. Aggressive student behavior is not nearly the conundrum it once was. Studies have provided new insights into the role of the family and the school in aggression development and maintenance, and this has led to promising research on effective organizational structures and programs for prevention at the primary, secondary, and tertiary levels. This book represents an effort to bridge the gap between that research and the school practitioners who need to put it to use.

In Chapter 1, an effort is made to dispel the notion that the most prevalent forms of violence in school—fighting and aggressive assault—are random and unpredictable. Aggressive behavior in the middle and high school settings is examined as an interaction between individual factors within the student and the external factors that make up the school environment. Many potentially aggressive students bring idiosyncratic dispositional attitudes about aggression, show varying levels of biased processing about the behavior of those around them, and move in and out of affective states over which they may have very little internal control. The external environment of the school provides a minute-to-minute setting that either increases or decreases the likelihood of an aggressive outburst. It is argued that both the internal readiness and skill of the student and the influential effects of the environment must be the targets of any potentially effective intervention.

In Chapter 2, the critical foundation for a schoolwide approach to the management of aggressive student behavior is discussed. A three-tiered organizational structure (e.g., Walker, Ramsey, & Gresham, 2004) in which all students receive prevention programming relative to their risk status is explained, and the essential role of behaviorally skilled students in the schoolwide effort is emphasized. Providing a setting that allows for this largest group of students to rise to their full potential as those who exemplify the behavioral expectations of the school community is an often overlooked component in an aggression management framework.

In Chapter 3, the rationale for anger management and behavioral skills training as an essential aspect of a schoolwide disciplinary framework is put forward. One of the major failings of traditional discipline plans as they attempt to address aggressive students is the assumption that the student has the skill to inhibit his or her aggression and will do so if threatened with a suspension or other aversive consequence. With a significant subset of students who engage in aggressive behavior, there is a need to move beyond an aversive-consequences-only plan and provide them with the skills that will allow the general discipline structure to mediate their behavior. Students who do not know how to control their anger and aggression cannot and should not be expected to do so unless someone teaches them how.

Chapter 4 addresses the process of screening and identifying those students who are in need of anger and aggression management skills training. In many schools there is an abundant supply of short-tempered, aggressive students and not an equivalent supply of available time or personnel to work with them. How do educators determine which students should receive this training? In this chapter an efficient, three-level needs hierarchy is proposed that makes use of existing data in the students' records to help school personnel reduce the potential for false positives and identify those students most likely to benefit.

Chapters 5 and 6 guide the practitioner through the practical "nuts and bolts" of preparing for and starting an anger and aggression skills-training intervention. Some of the critical issues that are covered include determining who does and does not need parental consent, building in generalization supports, specific adaptations for working with girls, and organizing a group behavior management strategy.

Finally, readers are presented with the complete treatment manual for the newly revised *Think First: Anger and Aggression Management for Secondary-Level Students*. This intervention is designed explicitly for the school setting, and the manual assists both novice and experienced counselors and school psychologists in implementing a research-supported, cognitive-behavioral intervention in a small-group format. Considerable effort has been made to organize the intervention in a practitioner-friendly format while adhering to evidence-supported treatment techniques. The manual is organized in a "module" format with identified learning outcomes that allows for flexibility to meet individual training needs. Abundant "Trainers' Hints," helpful forms, and useful student handouts assist the practitioner along the way. An optional supporting video is also available from the author.

Designing and implementing a schoolwide program to address the needs of middle school and high school students with problematic aggression is a serious undertaking that requires perseverance, attention to the research, and a sturdy self-concept. Students who are still adhering to anger-induced, aggressive conflict resolution strategies by the time they reach adolescence are a truly high-risk group. Their needs are many, and their behavior is extraordinarily difficult to change. When considering what to do, there are no panaceas, this book included.

As the literature makes clear, by the time young people reach middle school or high school it is frequently far too late to begin helping them manage problematic anger and aggression. That effort needs to have started years before. Angry, aggressive middle school students are statistically very likely to have been elementary-level students with serious problem behavior. If these problems were ignored, treated ineffectively, or merely contained as the child moved up the grades, then the secondary schools inherited the consequences. Whereas elementary educators know that second graders with reading problems will eventually become seventh graders with reading problems unless effective interventions are implemented, that same logic seems to escape them when it comes to problem behavior. This book strongly advocates the need for secondary personnel to take a K–12 perspective when it comes to addressing the needs of students with aggressive behavior. It can be said truthfully that the best friends of secondary-level educators are elementary educators who understand and implement evidence-supported prevention programming.

In closing, let me offer a "tip of the hat" to those practitioners who have made the decision to assertively address the needs of their students who exhibit problem aggression. If one takes the long view and measures this effort against the potential benefits for the students and for the society in which they will live, it is a reasonable, evidenced-based, and ethically sound decision. It is also one that I believe will never be regretted.

Acknowledgments

◆

This book is dedicated to my parents, Col. (Ret.) James D. Larson and Dorothy Larson, for their unending love and support. Their personal dedication to the value of hard work and perseverance in the face of life's challenges is a model for all their children. The book is also dedicated to my son, Jeremy, who teaches me daily about the strength and goodness alive in the youth of this world. In addition, I want to acknowledge the influence and work of my friends at the Melissa Institute for Violence Prevention and Treatment in Miami, Florida. This group of dedicated individuals, who turned a great tragedy—the murder of college student Melissa Aptman—into a remarkable and powerful force for good, reminds us all of what can happen with will, commitment, and endless heart. May your sunflowers forever be in bloom. Finally, I express my sincere thanks to Shirley Cottle, Allison Erickson, Katy Gunderson, and DeAnne Nuckles for their very kind assistance in the preparation of this book.

Contents

♦

THINK FIRST

CHAPTER 1

♦ ♦ ♦

The Problem and Directions for Change

♦

THE PROBLEM OF VIOLENCE IN THE SCHOOL SETTING

The school shootings that occurred in the United States in the late 1990s riveted Americans' attention on the issue of school violence. Unfortunately, and perhaps irrevocably, in some cases, the names of some of the communities where the shootings occurred have become associated with that difficult interlude: Pearl, Mississippi; West Paducah, Kentucky; Jonesboro, Arkansas; Springfield, Oregon; and Littleton, Colorado. Thirty-six students and teachers were killed during the period from 1996 to 2001 in student-perpetrated homicides that the U.S. Secret Service termed "targeted school violence" (Vossekuil, Fine, Reddy, Borum, & Modzeleski, 2002, p. 13).

Media attention to these crimes created a near panic situation as communities across the nation wondered and worried if their town would be in the next headline. Following the massacre at Columbine High School in 1999, a survey found that 71% of respondents believed that a school shooting was "likely" to occur in their community (Brooks, Schiraldi, & Zeidenberg, 2000). The facts were at odds with community perception, however. These authors concluded that even during the year of the Columbine shooting, the odds of a student dying in school was about 1 in 2 million. As shocking and tragic as these shootings were, national data have consistently demonstrated that homicide rates in the schools have shown a steady decrease since 1992 (National School Safety Center, 2003). Whereas only a foolish educator would dismiss even the possibility of homicidal violence in his or her building, it is clear that prevention energy and effort need to be directed elsewhere.

School violence takes many other forms beyond the rare homicide, and it is a very real problem. Along with the more obvious forms of physical aggression and illegal acts, the National Association of School Psychologists (2002) identified chronic bullying, name calling, sexual harassment, social exclusion, and mean-spirited teasing as forms of violence that threaten the psychological, physical, and emotional well-being of students and staff. For example, in a nationally representative sample of 15,686 students in the United States (grades 6–10), 29.9% reported frequent involvement in bullying at school, with 13% participating as bullies, 10.9% as victims, and 6% as both (Nansel et al., 2001). Related to bullying, the often devastating problems of social exclusion and peer rejection encountered principally by girls through relational and indirect aggression has been the subject of increasing study (Crick, 1996; Crick & Grotpeter, 1995; Crick et al., 2001). In addition, in a national survey of 2,064 public school students in 8th through 11th grades, it was found that approximately 83% of girls and 79% of boys reported that they had experienced sexual harassment at some point during their school years, with over 25% experiencing it "often" (American Association of University Women, 2001). Clearly, the public schools face many challenges in the effort to provide all students with a safe and supportive learning environment. One of the biggest challenges is to understand and intervene effectively with students who engage in chronic physical aggression.

Students who engage in overt, nonlethal physical aggression in school present a serious challenge to the maintenance of a safe and orderly learning environment. Unlike bullying and other less open forms of student behavior that are subsumed under school violence, fighting is explicit and violent, and it demands attention. A fight between students in a classroom, a hallway, or a lunchroom brings every other activity to a halt and draws fellow students and concerned adults toward the violence, both as onlookers and interveners. The disruption is total, the aftereffects lingering, and the potential for serious injury very real.

The fight seemed to come out of nowhere. The noisy high school lunchroom was packed as usual for first lunch at 11:40 A.M. Students were waiting in the hot lunch line, milling about around the tables, or already eating with their favorite group of companions.

The two teachers assigned to lunch duty were chatting together near the entrance door, checking identification cards as the late arrivals hurried in. This was a Monday, and, consequently, the two veteran staff members were alert for problems. "Weekend spillover," it was called; interpersonal student conflicts that started at parties and social settings over the weekend and got settled at school, too often with fists. The phenomenon was more occasional than it was regular, but the presence of an administrator walking about by the far wall indicated the level of extra preparedness.

A tall sophomore by the name of Jesse appeared at the entrance and showed his ID card.

"This is for second lunch, Jesse. You belong in class," said one of the teachers, inspecting the card.

"Yeah, I know, but I just gotta talk with somebody for a second. He's right over there."

The student pointed into the lunchroom, and as the teachers instinctively turned their heads, he bolted past them.

"Hey!"

Before anyone could make an intercepting move, the young man was into the lunchroom, pushing his way past other students, knocking a girl to the floor. Other students, recognizing the coming excitement, rose from their lunch tables as Jesse drew to a halt in front of another sophomore by the name of Michael. Michael stood to meet the challenge, but as he did, Jesse was all over him, fists flying.

Nearby students cheered on the combatants, encouraged by the excitement that was breaking up the monotony of another school day. The two boys tumbled into the salad bar as they pummeled one another, noses, lips, and shirts red with blood. Many from the noisy student audience climbed on the tables to get a better look. Pushing frantically past the crowd of onlookers, all three staff members and a helpful custodian eventually broke up the melee. The administrator sustained a sprained wrist for his troubles while escorting the two battered and angry students to the office.

Meanwhile, several blocks away at the middle school, Ms. Sara Chester was bringing her fourth-period eighth-grade general science class to order. It was a difficult class, due in part to both the age of the students and the fact that their reading skills varied by as much as five to six grade levels across the class. The competent, mostly serious students had to compete for teacher attention with their less able, more disruptive classmates. This was her first year teaching, and the enthusiastic, if yet unskilled, Ms. Chester found classroom management a challenge. Five minutes after the bell, the door opened and a stocky youth by the name of Jared appeared and headed for his seat, acknowledging the greetings of some pals.

"Whoa there, young man," said Ms. Chester. "Let's see that tardy pass."

The youth stopped by his desk and dug through his pockets with high drama while the class snickered.

"Must have lost it on the way," he said with an innocent shrug.

"Maybe it was flushed down the toilet with your cigarette," quipped Robert, a nearby classmate.

Jared turned to him, angrily. "Maybe I'll flush you down the toilet, ass-face!"

"Maybe you'll kiss my ass first." Robert stood, knocking his chair over.

"That's enough!" shouted Ms. Chester, now moving toward Jared, who hurled an obscenity at Robert.

The inexperienced teacher mistakenly moved to place herself between the two, holding her palms up to Jared and urging him to calm down. Jared spat out another loud obscenity over her shoulder, and the teacher suddenly felt the wind knocked from her as Robert attacked from behind. The girls screamed as they watched their teacher fall to the floor, the side of her head knocking against a desktop. One of the girls ran to the security button near the door and pressed it while some of the other boys attempted to pull Jared and Robert apart.

The current data regarding physical fighting among students is compelling. According to the National Center for Educational Statistics, in the year 2001, 33% of students in grades 9 through 12 reported that they had been in physical fights in the previous 12 months, and 13% reported that they had fought on school property. Although male students were more likely to have been in fights, 24% of female students reported that they had been in physical fights in the previous year and that 7% of this fighting took place on school property (DeVoe et al., 2002). Students are not the only ones to face the problem of physical violence in school. Over the 5-year period from 1996 through 2000, teachers were the victims of approximately 1,603,000 nonfatal crimes at school, including 1,004,000 thefts and 599,000 violent crimes involving rape or sexual assault, robbery, aggravated assault, and simple assault (DeVoe et al., 2002). A recent *New York Times* article noted that student assaults in New York City against teachers have risen by 26%, from 690 at the end of 2002 to 869 in 2003 (Herszenhorn, 2003). These alarming student and teacher statistics exist in the context of a generally declining number of some other school-violence-related behaviors (Brener, Simon, Krug, & Lowry, 1999). Whereas the number of homicides and weapon-carrying incidents in schools has followed a clear downward trajectory over the past decade, the prevalence of nonlethal assaults has remained fairly stable since the mid-1990s. Why is it that students continue to attack one another and their teachers?

To attempt to answer this question, Greene and his colleagues (Greene, Buka, Gortmaker, DeJong, & Winsten, 1997) from the Harvard School of Public Health surveyed a national sample of 1,558 middle and high school students in the United States in order to obtain their opinions about fighting. Sixty-six percent of these students reported having been in or witnessed a fight in the year prior to the survey. The students were asked to reflect on the most recently occurring fight in their memory and then to provide what they thought to be the reason for the conflict. These students provided the following:

Someone insulted someone else or treated them disrespectfully (54%).
There was an ongoing feud or disagreement (44%).
Someone was hit, pushed, shoved, or bumped (42%).
There were rumors or things people were saying (40%).
Someone could not control his or her anger (39%).
Other people were watching or encouraging the fight (34%).
Someone who likes to fight a lot was involved (26%).
Someone didn't want to look like a loser (21%).
There was an argument over a boyfriend or girlfriend (19%).
Someone wanted to keep a reputation or get a name (17%).

Interestingly, these researchers found that disputes involving illegal drugs or alcohol accounted for only 3% of the reasons for student fights.

The survey also asked the respondents to signify their agreement or disagreement with a number of statements. Thirty-three percent of the students agreed with the statement, "when I am really angry, there is no way I can control myself," and 41% agreed with the statement "If I am challenged, I am going to fight." These two endorsements exemplify what appear to be two firmly held belief structures among many adolescents across the aggressive behavior spectrum: (1) "I do not have control over my own level of anger because it is controlled by my antagonist, " and (2) "A challenge to fight means I must fight. There are no personally acceptable alternatives." An individual who believes that the locus of control for his or her anger lies exclusively with someone else is highly likely to aggress against that person to obtain anger relief. In effect, the conclusion is, "I have to hit you so that you will stop making me angry."

The second belief structure that demands an aggressive response to any challenge to fight is deeply rooted among many in the youth culture and modeled repeatedly in movies and television programs directed at young people. When I was a school psychologist serving a large high school, an oft-repeated justification from the fighters was, "My father told me not to start nothin', but don't take no shit from nobody either," or "My mama said if anybody disrespects our family, you hit 'em." Whereas the actual *saying* of these admonitions by the real fathers and mothers was almost surely apocryphal, the message of "never back down from a challenge of any kind" was pervasive across the culture of young fighters.

The respondents in the Greene et al. (1997) survey were "typical" middle and high school students, not necessarily the individuals whose problematic fighting behavior is the subject of this volume. Yet their perspective is not so different from that of their more aggressive peers. One of the most comprehensive studies of adolescent fighting behavior from the perspective of the individuals who were directly involved was completed by Lockwood (1997). For this study, the researchers interviewed students in a middle school located in an economically disadvantaged section of a major urban area in the southern United States and high school students from a large Midwestern city who had been administratively placed in an alternative school setting for disciplinary reasons. The subject pool consisted of 70 boys and 40 girls. The author noted that the subject pool was highly skewed toward individuals most likely to stand a chance of becoming involved in violence and was not representative of the general population of middle and high school students:

The interviews were open-ended, with the students encouraged to speak at length about the violent incidents in which they had been involved. A total of 250 "incidents," most taking place within the past year, came to light in the interviews. The conversations explored the dynamics of the incidents from the perspective of the young people and were concerned with behavior, emotions, values, and attitudes at different steps of the violent encounter. The researchers examined such factors as goals, excuses, and justifications for the incidents. (Lockwood, 1997, p. 4)

Some of the key findings from this research were the following:

- The average number of violent incidents experienced by the girls was nearly the same as that experienced by the boys. Girls were equally as likely to fight with boys as with other girls.
- Of the incidents that occurred in school, about half took place in the classroom, with the remainder in other supervised areas, including the gym.
- The most common role of peers was to encourage or join in the fight. In only 3% of the incidents did peers attempt to mediate the conflict.
- The most frequently cited goals of the violent behavior were retribution (40% of all goals), compliance demands (22%), self- or other defense (21%), and image promotion/reputation management (8%).
- The conflicts contained "working agreements" (p. 6) in which a youth invited or challenged another youth to fight, and the challenge was accepted. In nearly two-thirds of the incidents, such invitations preceded the actual physical altercation.
- The feeling of anger was experienced by 62% of the students involved in the incidents, whereas only 14% described experiencing fear.
- In 84% of the incident accounts, the combatants accepted responsibility for their aggressive behavior but denied that their actions were wrong. In most cases, the students who initiated the aggression said that the victim had done something to deserve it.

A common element in most of the incidents was what the author described as an *opening move,* defined as "the action of the student, the student antagonist, or third party that initiates the violent incident" (Lockwood, 1997, p. 6). In 70% of the cases, the students ascribed the opening move to someone else, not themselves. However, in less than 10% percent of the incidents were the actions following this opening move intended to avoid the fight through retreat or any other means.

THE CONTEXT OF SCHOOL-BASED AGGRESSIVE BEHAVIOR

What can school personnel do to address this problem? The answer is complex and requires an examination of the major environmental and personal interactions that set the stage for physical aggression in the school context. The contextual characteristics of the school environment, the cognitive-emotional characteristics and skills of the individuals involved, and the seemingly entrenched values and belief systems of highly aggressive youths all contribute. Let us turn first to the setting—the general population of students interacting within a defined space—and examine its potential influence on aggressive student behavior.

Who's in School?

Approximately 14 million students attend middle and high schools in the United States. When attempting to understand the challenges inherent in providing a meaningful and safe educational experience for all students, it is useful to examine who is in school and who is not. According to the National Center for Educational Statistics (2001):

> Public school enrollment in kindergarten through grade eight rose from 29.9 million in fall 1990 to an estimated 33.6 million in fall 2001. Enrollment in the upper grades rose from 11.3 million in 1990 to 13.6 million in 2001. The growing numbers of young pupils that have been filling the elementary schools will cause some increases at the secondary school level during the next 10 years. Between fall 2001 and fall 2011, public elementary enrollment is expected to remain fairly stable, while public secondary school enrollment is expected to rise by 3 percent. Public school enrollment is projected to set new records every year until 2005. (Enrollment trends, public and private schools section)

Everyone in this country has a right to a free and appropriate public education, regardless of any disabling, ethnic, family, behavioral, or socioeconomic characteristic. If they show up, they have the right to expect to be included in the general curriculum to the extent possible. Moreover, the courts have decided that education officials may not interrupt or terminate those rights just because the student is unable or unwilling to adhere to the rules of the school or community. I recall an incident that happened once when I was home visiting my parents. My father, a retired Air Force officer, needed to go to my younger brother's high school to deliver some forgotten homework. When he returned, he was livid with anger:

> "You would not believe what is going on in that school! Slovenly dressed hoodlums standing around smoking cigarettes outside, couples necking in the parking lot, hallways full of half-dressed girls and pink-haired boys cursing aloud and fondling each other! I cannot believe it! That's a school? In my day, the principal would have simply said, 'Shape up or ship out,' and, believe me, they would, or they would have been gone in a heartbeat! Here's the door. Don't come back."

Of course, he was right on that last count. American public high schools in the first half of the 20th century existed, if not exclusively, primarily for students whom the schools were ready and willing to educate. If students did not have the ability to keep up, if they had some manner of disabling condition, if they disobeyed the rules of behavior, or if they simply rubbed some administrator the wrong way, they could be simply erased from the rolls. No paperwork in triplicate, no due process hearings, no lawyers. Those who were left in school were the students whom my father recalled from his day: academically competent, obedient of school rules, respectful to adults, and generally serious about their educations.

Then again, the overall high school graduation rate in 1950 was less than 50% ("Dropout Rates in the United States," 1996). One might rejoin that much of the labor force of that time did not require a high school diploma, and that is correct. Many of those who chose to leave school or were barred from attending found steady and often lucrative employment—that is, those without seriously disabling conditions or "undesirable" racial or ethnic characteristics. The bleak specters of discrimination and racism were, of course, very much a part of the education and labor scenes during the "good old days."

The 14th Amendment and the Arrival of Diversity

In 1961, when I was in the seventh grade, the Air Force transferred my father to Robbins Air Force Base, located outside of Macon, Georgia. It was my family's first posting in the Deep South, and it was an eye-opener. Because no on-base housing was available to us at that time, we secured a home in the city of Macon. I grew up in the comparatively integrated world of the military, so I was intellectually and emotionally unprepared for what Macon had to offer in 1963. I enrolled at Sydney Lanier Junior High School, a school that was segregated not only by race but also by gender. At the junior and senior high school levels, all of the white boys went to one school, and all of the white girls went to another. The African American students went to different schools from kindergarten through high school. For a student in Macon at that time, there was literally no contact between the races that was officially sanctioned by the school district.

The population in the hallways and classrooms of American public schools in almost any city, including Macon, look very much different today. Racial diversity where there once was legal segregation and ramps where there once were only stairways are two of the most prominent indicators of that difference. Over the past nearly five decades, the courts have concluded that schools must provide equal educational opportunities for all children. The 14th Amendment of the Constitution contains the *equal protection clause* that provides that no state shall "deny any person within its jurisdiction the equal protection of the laws." In particular, rulings that culminated in the landmark 1954 decision in *Brown v. Board of Education* established that states must provide equal education to all children regardless of race. This decision has since been extended to issues of national origin, native language, sex, and handicapping condition (Jacob & Hartshorne, 2003). Although racial integration of American public schools has come with an enormous share of tumult, pain, and de facto discrimination, and although it has ongoing and serious issues yet to address, *Brown* changed the landscape of education forever. Few today would argue against the "rightness" of racially equal educational opportunities in a democratic society.

The 14th Amendment to the Constitution holds that no state shall "deprive any person of life, liberty, *or property*, without due process of law" (emphasis added). Ruling in the 1975 *Goss v. Lopez* case, the Supreme Court held that to deprive an individual of an education is to deprive that individual of a property right (Jacob & Hartshorne, 2003). Barring or otherwise excluding any individual from a free and appropriate public education was determined to be akin to relieving that individual of some other manner of legally owned property and, consequently, could not be accomplished without some form of legal due process. Students had rights, and those rights had to be protected. The days of casually excluding misbehaving, underachieving, or otherwise less than desirable students were not over after *Goss* by any means, but a significant impediment had been added that would forever change the day-to-day population of American public schools.

The 14th Amendment also provides the constitutional foundation for an additional landmark piece of legislation that further helps answer the question, "Who is in school?" That legislation is Public Law 94-142, the Education of All Handicapped Children Act of 1975 (now Public Law 105-17, the Individuals with Disabilities Education Act Amendments of 1997, known as IDEA). IDEA provides funds to states and localities to provide a free and appropriate public education to all children with disabilities in accordance with the requirements of the law (Jacob & Hartshorne, 2003). Under IDEA, a child with a disability means a child who has met the evaluation and program criteria for

> mental retardation, hearing impairments (including deafness), speech or language impairments, visual impairments (including blindness), serious emotional disturbance (hereafter referred to as "emotional disturbance"), orthopedic impairments, autism, traumatic brain injury, other health impairments, or specific learning disabilities; and . . . who, by reason thereof, needs special education and related services. (Pub. L. No. 105-17, §602, 111 Stat. 43 [1997])

In the 1999–2000 school year, the number of students ages 6 through 21 with disabilities who were served under Part B of IDEA reached 5,683,707, a 2.6% increase over the 1998–1999 school year (Office of Special Education Programs, 2001). With IDEA came the principle of *zero reject*. This principle means that the states must provide full educational opportunities to all children with disabilities, regardless of the severity of their disabilities (Jacob & Hartshorne, 2003). No child with a disability—be it cognitive, physical, or emotional–behavioral—can be so impaired that he or she does not have the right to a free and appropriate public education in the company of nondisabled peers to the extent possible. Whether that child demonstrates that he or she is willing or able to benefit from special education is irrelevant; services must be provided.

It has become abundantly clear over the years that the inclusion of all students into the fabric of American schools is proper not only from a legal standpoint but also from moral and educational standpoints. When diversity in the public schools mirrors or even exceeds that of the greater society, all students have the opportunity to benefit from the coeducational experiences. Students without disabilities who qualify under IDEA have opportunities to befriend and learn in the company of students who do have such disabilities. The resulting inclusion can promote relationships with the general education students that move beyond passive acceptance of students with disabilities to active understanding and shared commitments to one another's well-being.

In the 1999–2000 school year, 470,111 students with emotional–behavioral disabilities (EBD) were served in the public schools under IDEA, approximately 20% more than a decade earlier (Office of Special Education Programs, 2001). Students with these disabilities are often at very high risk for comorbid antisocial behavior patterns (Walker, 1993) and persistent, often aggressive, problem behavior that lead to frequent disciplinary encounters. Students with EBD are also at very high risk for personal victimization. Doren, Bullis, and Benz (1996) found that students who were classified as EBD were 20.48 times more likely than nondisabled peers to experience victimization while in school. Not surprisingly, of all the special education categories of student disabilities, students with EBD have the highest school dropout rate, approaching nearly 50% (Office of Special Education Programs, 2001).

The student population in today's public schools is also defined by increased racial and ethnic diversification. From 1986 to 1999, the percentage of nonwhite students (black, Hispanic, Asian, or Native American) increased 29.7% of all students to 38% (National Center for Educational Statistics, 2001). A measure of how well the public school system has responded to these changes may be seen in school dropout percentages. If all of the students between the ages of 16 and 24 who did not finish high school and did not go on to obtain the generalized equivalency diploma (GED) are examined for that same period, the results indicate a problem. The school dropout rate among Hispanic males remained *relatively constant* at slightly over 30%, and among black males at slightly over 15%. The dropout rate among white male students *fell* from 10.3% in 1986 to 7.7% in 1999 (National Center for Educational Statistics, 2001). These data clearly indicate that the United States public school system is not meeting the educational needs of a significant portion of its student body. Additionally, the data indicate that larger and larger numbers of poorly skilled, poorly educated minority individuals are somewhere other than in the school building between the hours of 8 A.M. and 4 P.M. on a daily basis.

The beginning of this millennium finds the public secondary schools characterized by diversity in all its iterations—color, academic proficiency, disabling condition, behavior management skills, political and social perspective, sexual orientation, and socioeconomic status. Some schools have more of one and less of another, but the dehomogenizing of the nation's public schools is a fact of life and one that comes equipped with its own set of challenges.

The Physical Setting for Aggressive Behavior

Indulge in a bit of whimsy for a minute. Let's say that there was a society in which every man, woman, and child was allowed to do exactly what he or she wanted to do, all the time. They could work or not work at their pleasure, play when they wanted to play, and all were equally free to do whatever their hearts desired. And let's further say that everything in this imaginary society was working out very well. The inhabitants were happy, content, and free from conflict.

Now consider this. What if the members of this society decided that they had become bored with all this contentment and actually wanted to infuse stress and conflict into this society? A very good way to go about doing it would be to start with the most potentially volatile of their numbers, the adolescents.

Here's the plan: This society will now require that all young people between the ages of 11 and 18 be rounded up early in the morning against their wills and sent to a stark, cold building full of hard chairs and desks. There they will be forced to remain for 7 hours, obeying rules that they had no say in making and performing tasks that they would otherwise not choose to do. Every 50 minutes or so, they will be forced to leave one room and make their way through a common hallway to another room, where they will once again be forced to engage in an aversive task.

There will now be a large aggregation of intellectually, behaviorally, and academically diverse teenagers engaging in personally unselected and, by and large, undesired behaviors generally against their collective will in an environment of limited space. Is there any chance for stress and conflict now?

Whimsy aside, the notion that the often peculiar nature of a typical school building environment is a contributing factor to the problem behavior found within is worthy of serious examination. The National Research Council (1993) observed:

> Spatial characteristics of school can influence violence in that (a) relatively high numbers of individuals occupy a limited amount of space, (b) the imposition of behavioral routines and conformity may contribute to feelings of anger, resentment, and rejection, and (c) poor design features may facilitate the commission of violent acts. (p. 371)

The vast majority of young people are able to negotiate their middle and high school years without engaging in violent physical confrontations in the school setting or, for that matter, in any other setting. Regardless of the age, size, or other features of their school buildings, they show up, participate, and eventually move on to postsecondary activities. For these students, consideration of the context of school is relevant primarily to the quality of their academic opportunities. For instance, recent studies report that small and moderate-sized secondary schools promote greater learning opportunities for economically disadvantaged students, and that, overall, students in moderate-sized schools (600–900 students) have the greatest learning opportunities (National Center for Educational Statistics, 2003). When the focus is on young people at risk for physical aggression, however, a closer examination of the context is essential to understanding.

Setting Events and Aggressive Behavior

Behaviorists refer to the context, conditions, or other characteristics of external physical environments and internal personal states that influence the likelihood or set the stage for certain behaviors as *setting events* (Kazdin, 2001). Setting events do not *cause* a behavior to occur; rather, they serve to increase or decrease the *probability* that a particular behavior will occur.

Feelings of irritability, frustration, lack of sleep, medication status, or even hunger are all examples of *internal* setting events in that they increase the probability for some behaviors. One spouse may say to the other:

"I'm sorry. I'm just frustrated with this project. I didn't mean to snap at you."

In this case, the internal setting event of frustration set the stage for "snap at you" behavior, behavior that might be a low probability in other circumstances. Similarly, a youth who comes to school upset after an emotional argument with his or her parents (internal setting event) may be at increased risk for atypical behaviors, such as distractibility or even impulsive anger outbursts. The student's emotional upset cannot be considered the cause of the school behaviors, but it can be seen as increasing the probability that those behaviors will emerge.

External setting events involve the features of immediate physical environment, the behavior of others in that environment, and the nature of the task or demand presented to the individual (Kazdin, 2001). The presence of a police car with its radar on in the median (external setting event) does not cause drivers to slow down, but it certainly increases the likelihood that they will. The probability of speeding in that context is decreased, and the probability of slower driving is increased. Importantly, however, the actual choice to enact the behavior of slowing down still remains with the driver.

Most of us are aware of other kinds of efforts to influence our behavior by the systematic altering of our environments to increase the probability of some behavior or feeling state. In the commercial world, architects, geographers, psychologists, and others collaborate to design settings to maximize potential for desired behaviors in a particular circumstance. For example, the use of large, "anchor" department stores located at opposite ends of a shopping center is designed to increase the likelihood that shoppers will visit smaller shops on their journey from one to the other. Disney

World, in Orlando, Florida, is an excellent example of the interaction of human engineering psychology and architectural creativity. The planners who created Disney World knew that success would be built on their ability to create an environment that increased the likelihood of safe, orderly, pleasure-seeking behavior, even in a crowded park when the temperature was 95 degrees. As an example:

> There are only three buildings on Main Street that are full scale: Welcome Center, Train Station and City Hall. The others are gradually done to a smaller scale as you work your way up Main Street to the Castle. This is done to make it look like the Castle is bigger than it is as you go in to the park, and as you leave dead tired, the Train Station looks closer than it really is. ("Disney Fun Facts," 2003, General section)

The student's day in a public school building is composed of a variety of external setting events ostensibly organized to increase the likelihood of safe, orderly, learning behavior. A classroom is an external setting event that has been designed to increase the likelihood that sitting, listening, and writing behavior will occur. (Whether any of these behaviors results in learning may be a separate issue.) Alternately, a gymnasium is a setting event that sets the stage for the potential for more robust physical activity. A hallway is a setting event designed to increase the probability of efficient movement from one location to another. Students find themselves in a variety of these environmental conditions during the course of a school day and select behaviors from among their repertoire that they believe to be in their best interest in that context.

The physical characteristics of the setting have a varying influence on the student's choice of behavior. The observed presence of the police liaison officer or school security officials in a crowded entryway may increase the likelihood that nonaggressive behaviors will be enacted by students in that context. A long lecture in an overly warm, poorly lit classroom encountered at the end of the school day can increase the probability of nonacademically oriented behaviors, such as daydreaming and doodling (an experience familiar to most of us). It is important to note that both of these conditions do not guarantee such behaviors; they only increase their probability. In both scenarios any individual may select an alternative behavior. In spite of the presence of the police, an angry student may still aggress against another, and an academically motivated student may hang on every word of the lecture. Understanding the power of setting events to influence behavior also means recognizing the futility of perfect prediction. Even Disney World has its share of unhappy visitors.

The Interaction of External and Internal Setting Events

External and internal setting events interact and have a major influence on selected behaviors. Most of us can recall instances in which a previously fun or relaxing activity was not fun or relaxing because of something bothersome on our minds. On a beautiful evening you may sit outside on your deck with a friend and a cool beverage, but you can't seem to enjoy it as you usually do because of worry about getting the results from a recent physical examination. The family Thanksgiving dinner, historically a setting event that increased the likelihood of joy and festive behavior, produces neither because of the argument you had in the car on the way over. In both these examples, the external setting events set the stage for some high-probability behaviors, but they interacted with a temporary internal setting event. Consequently, those high probability behaviors were not enacted.

Consider the external setting event of a crowded high school hallway during passing time. A 16-year-old junior named Jeremy with no history of aggressive behavior gets jostled just after an angry run-in with his girlfriend (internal setting event). Whereas on most other days he would ignore it and continue to his next class, he reacts uncharacteristically with an aggressive response, shoving the offending student to the floor. A fight ensues. Such interactions of transient mood and environment are generally unpredictable and are typically viewed as the cost of doing business with large groups of adolescents. School personnel obviously cannot plan for every possible contingency and must instead react to each one on an incident-by-incident basis.

Setting Events and Implications for Interventions

Although the random clashes between external setting events and the temporary internal state of any particular student are difficult to anticipate, for some students plans for just such contingencies may be built into their programs. For years teachers, school psychologists, and other professionals who work with special education students have known of the need to make modifications in the school environment to accommodate the often unique behavioral, cognitive, and emotional qualities of their students. These modifications are referred to as positive behavioral supports (PBS; see Carr et al., 1999, for a review).

In the school setting, PBS alter the setting events encountered by a specific individual so as to increase the likelihood of desired behaviors. They are the efforts of informed and responsible others to make the student's environment most conducive to his or her abilities to select the desired behavior. As O'Neill et al. (1997) point out:

> Plans of behavior support define what we will do differently. It is the change in our behavior that will result in improved behavior of the focus person. The plan may involve changes we will make in the physical setting, changes in curriculum, changes in the medications we will administer, changes in schedule, changes in how we teach, and changes in rewards and punishers. A good behavior support plan defines in very specific detail the changes expected in the behavior of relevant teachers, family members, or staff. (p. 65)

Consider a young man in high school with severe and chronic anger control problems who receives services under the IDEA for students with EBD. This young person may have an Individualized Education Plan (IEP) that structures his day in such a manner that the predictable setting events that occasion his anger outbursts are replaced with those that increase the probability of more controlled emotions. Altered passing times, low-student-density classrooms, settings and opportunities for quiet time, shortened school days, and curriculum matched to his abilities may all be put in place to provide him the behavioral support he needs to minimize the potential for anger outbursts. Pursuing their quests to increase the likelihood of nonviolent conflict resolution among all students, general education professionals can learn from the experience and research acquired by special educators in the uses of PBS. Further discussion of how this may be accomplished is found in Chapter 2.

In the effort to understand the complexities that set the stage for physical aggression in the school context, I have shown how internal and external setting events, individually and in interaction, can influence a student's choice of behavior. Some school settings and some transient emotional circumstances increase the potential for physically aggressive behavior. Let us now look more carefully at the individual students themselves.

Clearly, there are some students who fight more than others, who just seem to attract trouble, and who seem uncommonly resistant to school disciplinary responses. They are the regular denizens of the discipline administrator's waiting area. They challenge the teacher's authority and ignore their class work. They threaten, shove, and fight in the hallways. They populate the weekend detention programs and the alternative schoolhouses. They are often out on the streets or home in bed when their peers are in school. They show up in numbers in the 9th grade and have vanished well before the 12th.

Across the country in rural and urban schools alike, there are students attending on a daily basis who possess cognitive, emotional, and behavioral repertoires that actually make avoiding a fight or some other physical altercation extremely difficult for them. Prevalent among such students are those who have been described in the literature as having *social-cognitive deficits*—predominantly learned, cognitive-behavioral patterns that alter and limit the manner in which they perceive, process, and react to certain environmental stimuli. Let us now explore who these individuals are.

SOCIAL-COGNITIVE DEFICITS AND PHYSICAL AGGRESSION

Much of the research that attempts to understand how highly aggressive children and youths process information and make behavioral decisions has been done by Kenneth Dodge, John Lochman, and their colleagues (see Larson & Lochman, 2002, and

Lochman, Whidby, & FitzGerald, 2000, for reviews). Dodge and his colleagues (e.g., Crick & Dodge, 1994; Dodge, 1991; Dodge, Pettit, McClaskey, & Brown, 1986) conceptualized a social information-processing model of anger arousal and aggressive behavior that has been highly influential in the understanding of aggressive reactions. The model draws on social learning theory, attribution theory, and decision-making theory in its effort to explain aggressive behavior. As Pettit (1997) noted:

> Social information processing describes the cognitive processes involved in an individual's response to a specific social situation. Of particular importance is an understanding of how individuals perceive social cues, make attributions and inferences about those cues, generate solutions to social dilemmas or problems, and make behavioral decisions about how to respond to those problems (including decisions whether or not to aggress). (pp. 141–142)

In the social information-processing model, Dodge and his colleagues identified six cognitive steps that an individual utilizes to process social information. The steps are as follows:

1. Encoding of social cues in the immediate environment.
2. Interpreting the meaning of those cues.
3. Identifying personal goals or desired outcomes.
4. Generating possible behavioral responses to the interpreted cues.
5. Deciding on a response and evaluating its potential outcome.
6. Engaging in the selected behavior

It is important to understand that, although there appears to be a linear flow, with discrete "steps," in actuality the processes are more parallel than sequential. As Crick and Dodge (1994) observed:

> Undoubtedly, individuals are engaged in multiple social information-processing activities at the same time (e.g., they engage in interpretation processes while they are encoding cues, and they continue to consider the meaning of another's behavior while they access responses). It is probably more accurate to posit that, during all waking hours, individuals are perpetually engaging in each of the steps of processing proposed. So children are always encoding, interpreting, and accessing responses. (p. 77)

The encoding process (Step 1) occurs when an individual becomes aware, through sensory activation, of stimuli in his or her immediate environment. Simply put, the individual sees, hears, smells, or feels something and chooses to attend to it. The research on this model has demonstrated that an aggressive student will selectively attend to aggressive cues at higher rates than do those who are nonaggressive (Lochman et al., 2000). Whereas a nonaggressive eighth-grade basketball player might feel the pain of (encode) an elbow in the back, he is more likely than a highly aggressive player to immediately redirect his attention to more game-related information and play on. In contrast, a player with problematic aggression is more likely to find that elbow-in-the-back cue highly salient and focus his attention on it to the exclusion of additional cues and information. Anyone who has watched the NBA knows that such behavior is not limited to the eighth graders.

Imagine, for instance, that a highly aggressive, behaviorally problematic ninth-grade youth whom we shall call James is milling about the school entrance corridor with his friends before the start of classes, showing off his new cell phone. There is considerable student traffic entering the building, and there is the typical amount of loudness and adolescent jocularity. The social information-processing model posits that James will be hypervigilant for aggressive cues in his immediate environment— any word or deed by a peer that signals hostility or potential aggression. In the crowded student traffic, someone knocks the cell phone from James's hand, and it clatters to the floor.

The typical, nonaggressive student would most likely attend first to the cues that give him or her information about the safety of the new cell phone and immediately start to look for it on the floor. James, on the other hand, with his highly aggressive behavioral repertoire, attends first to the potential hostility of the person responsible for the incident, ignoring cues more typically relevant to the immediate situation. His eyes are up and scanning, not down and searching.

In Step 2, after the individual has selected the cue to which to attend (i.e., encoded it), he or she needs to give meaning to it by mental representation and interpretation (Dodge, 1991). This is a potentially complex and very critical step, for it has major implications for the direction that the steps to come will take. At this step the individual instantaneously searches his or her experiential memory for his or her own set of internalized interpretation rules to help in the accurate and meaningful representation of the encoded cues (Pettit, 1997). In other words, an individual's life experiences with cues similar to the one encoded have allowed him or her to make some generalizations about its meaning, and there is an attempt to fit the present situation into those generalized meanings. Our aggressive student, James, upon encoding the bump that knocked his cell phone to the floor, instantaneously has to decide whether *this bump* belongs in the category of *accidental bumps* or *hostile bumps*, for each has meaning. Highly aggressive youths are much more likely than their less aggressive counterparts to infer hostility in others (Dodge, Price, Bachorowski, & Newman, 1990). This inclination is what is known as a *hostile attributional bias*, or "the tendency to 'assume the worst' regarding the intention of peers in ambiguous (neither hostile nor benign) situations" (Kendall, Ronan, & Epps, 1991, p. 345). As he does in this instance, James habitually assumes the worst in many such ambiguous encounters with peers or staff members. In fact, he is so quick to do so and so disinclined to consider an alternative explanation such as an accident that his peers have learned to retaliate with equal habit and speed. Such peer retaliation has the effect of confirming his original hostile bias. It is a self-confirming circle of biased interpretation, hostile retaliation, and confirmation of the original hostile intent. He confronts his perceived assailant.

"Hey, asshole! What's up with trashing my cell phone?"
"Hey, screw you! I didn't trash no cell phone!"

They are chest to chest in the time-honored pose of male aggressive posturing. Step 3 in the social-information-processing model involves selecting a goal or a desired outcome. Such goals may include staying out of trouble, making a friend, getting even with a provocateur, or obtaining some material object (Crick & Dodge, 1994). The goal selection is highly related to the level of emotional arousal. Aggressive behavior has been conceptualized as being in part due to an inability to regulate emotional responses to anger-producing stimuli (Lochman, Dunn, & Wagner, 1997). If a youth interprets an ambiguous event as hostile (Step 2), he or she is likely to experience a surge of anger at a physiological level (Larson & Lochman, 2002). In the case of aggressive youths, that emotional arousal will influence goal selection (Step 3) in a meaningful way. In the case of James, his biased interpretation of hostility has fueled his anger, and his goals are clearly to get even with his perceived provocateur.

Now highly aroused with anger and aware of his goal, James enters Step 4 of the social information-processing model. At this juncture, it is hypothesized that individuals "access from memory possible responses to the situation, or, if the situation is novel, they may construct new behaviors in response to immediate social cues" (Crick & Dodge, 1994, p. 76). Simply put, they try to decide what to do now to achieve their goal. Research with aggressive children has demonstrated that they have both quantitative and qualitative deficiencies in the generation of problem-solving solutions (Lochman, Meyer, Rabiner, & White, 1991). Aggressive children and youths tend to generate more aggressive responses at the expense of verbal assertion solutions or compromise solutions (Larson & Lochman, 2002). It is hypothesized that this tendency is due to the lack of knowledge of nonaggressive responses (i.e., no one ever told them about such responses), lack of motivation to demonstrate the response (Pettit, 1997), or the saliency of their preference for direct action responses (Lochman & Lampron, 1986). In addition, the most severely aggressive and violent youths have a deficiency in the number of solutions they can generate to resolve social problems (Lochman & Dodge, 1994). In the example with James, this is a familiar situation in which he has found himself, and the only solutions he considers are aggressive ones. Although he may have understanding at a simple knowledge level of other, less aggressive responses, he has never tried them in similar situations and has no experience of them ever being functional for him. Chances are great, therefore, that he does not know how to enact them, and, consequently, they are not even considered. It is more likely that he is only considering aggressive variations, for example, more verbal accusations or threats, a shove, or a punch.

At Step 5 in this model, it is hypothesized that individuals evaluate the potential for positive outcomes in each of the constructed responses to the situation in order to select the one for enactment. In this task, individuals will consider factors such as confidence in their own ability to actually enact the behavior (Crick & Dodge, 1994). Although an aggressive youth may consider the possibility of a nonaggressive response, he or she will quickly dismiss it if confidence in the ability to carry it out to desirable outcome is absent. Like many highly aggressive youths, James has abundant confidence in his ability to enact an aggressive response. Experience has made him familiar with the behavior, he has trust in his skill to carry it out, and it has worked for him in the past in similar situations. In Step 6, he enacts the selected behavior and punches the other youth in the mouth. Another fight is on.

Social Information-Processing and Implications for Intervention

"Garbage in, garbage out" is an old computer programmers' saying that reflects a central principle in computer-based data input. The end product is only as good as the data that preceded it and upon which it is built. Enter faulty data at any point, and the subsequent entries that rely on those data will also be faulty. A similar analogy may be applied to humans who engage in faulty or biased encoding and processing of environmental stimuli. Many of us have had the experience of seeing or hearing something (e.g., emotionally loaded words in partially overheard conversation or a familiar face out of place in a passing car) and have acted on that "information" only to find out later that the data were faulty.

> "I heard you telling him that I was 'in over my head' or something like that."
> "At 1 P.M., you are supposed to be in school, not riding around in a car with some punk!"

With luck the behavior that arose out of the misperception was only temporarily embarrassing and perhaps brought on a vow to be more careful before jumping to conclusions in the future. Highly aggressive youths—those who exhibit chronic distortions and deficits in the manner in which they encode and process social information *on a regular basis*—experience much more than temporary embarrassment and seldom ever vow to be more careful. For these youths, the "garbage in" can eventually become "violence out."

When considering the training needs of physically aggressive youths from a cognitive-behavioral perspective, it is useful to hypothesize the possibility of biased or deficient processing at any point in the social encounter and to target that point for intervention. The social information-processing model offers the potential for intervention at any of the "steps" in the sequence.

Following a comprehensive assessment of the processing skills and deficits of the adolescent (see Chapter 4), a profile that targets training needs can be developed. For example, at Steps 1 and 2, is the adolescent able to acquire more effective encoding skills so as to decrease focus on the purely provocative aspects of the encounter, and does the adolescent have particular difficulty interpreting peers' intentions in provocative situations? Does the adolescent have the kind of hostile attributional bias that increases the likelihood that he or she will respond aggressively in ambiguous or potentially provocative situations? Initial work with this cognitive mechanism has been promising. Hudley and her colleagues (Hudley, 1992; Hudley et al., 1998) have shown positive results with an attribution-retraining program that targeted the biased attributions of aggressive African American boys of elementary-school age. These researchers devised an attribution-retraining program that they named "Brain-Power" and implemented it in four elementary schools. Over a period of 12 sessions, the students who had been identified as aggressive were trained to recognize alternative explanations for various interactions with peers. In addition, they discussed how to respond appropriately, without aggression, to such interactions. At the end of the program, the students who received the training were found to be less likely to make judgments of hostile intent than were students in a control group. Follow-up assessments in the following year of the boys who had received the BrainPower program indicated a significant drop-off in previous gains. The researchers noted that longer term effects may require that attribution retraining be integrated into a more comprehensive training program.

At Step 3, interventions must concentrate on helping the aggressive youths understand and accept the value of less aggressive and more prosocial goals in provocative peer encounters. An adolescent who has experienced chronic peer rejection may have surrendered all hope of acceptance goals and now may focus exclusively on fear-producing goals—that is, "If you won't like me, I'll make you respect me physically." Goldstein and colleagues (Goldstein, Glick, & Gibbs, 1998; Goldstein, Glick, Reiner, Zimmerman, & Coultry, 1986) used goal development as an integral part of their comprehensive program, Aggression Replacement Training, in their work with institutionalized delinquents.

It is at this step that Crick and Dodge (1994) also noted that arousal state has a significant influence upon goal selection and later problem-solving efficacy. Aggressive individuals are much more likely than their nonaggressive peers to label affect-arousing situations as producing anger rather than some other emotion, such as sadness (Lochman, White, & Wayland, 1991). A youth who responds to a provocation with high levels of anger is at a considerable disadvantage when attempting any effort to control an aggressive response. As Feindler and Scalley (1998) pointed out, "although aggression can certainly occur in the absence of anger arousal, theorists generally agree that anger can act as a determinant of aggressive behavior and will influence the cognitive processes used to mediate one's response to a perceived provocation" (p. 104). Individuals who are highly aroused with anger do not process information effectively and tend to be impulsive in their decision making and behavior. Although not all aggressive students have anger control problems, it is generally true that those students who do have significant anger problems also have co-occurring problems with some form of aggression. Clearly, anger management is an essential component in any cognitive-behavioral intervention with aggressive youth.

At Steps 4 and 5 in the social information processing model, the youth is in the process of making decisions about what behavior is in his or her best interest, and interventions must concentrate on providing the problem-solving skills necessary to perform this cognitive task more effectively. Numerous models exist to guide practitioners in this endeavor (e.g., D'Zurilla & Nezu, 1999; Meichenbaum, 2001). Typical problem-solving models utilize a process that reframes the threat or provocation as a problem to be solved (Meichenbaum, 2001) and teach the individuals to engage in a series of steps framed as questions:

1. What is the problem?
2. What are some possible solutions?
3. What are the probable consequences of each solution?
4. Which one will I select?
5. (Afterward) How did I do?

As noted, aggressive individuals demonstrate deficiencies in both the quantity and the quality of their problem-solving solutions (see Lochman, Meyer, et al., 1991). Training from a cognitive-behavioral orientation can provide the youth with contextually safe opportunities to practice response generation through simulated provocations. For example:

TRAINER: Let's say another student comes by and shuts your locker while you are looking for a book. What could you do?

YOUTH: I could smack him upside his head!

TRAINER: Yes, what else could you do?

YOUTH: Drag him back, and make him open it again.

TRAINER: Yes, you could do that, too. What could you do if you did not want to get physical with the other student in order to avoid a suspension?

YOUTH: Just ignore it?

TRAINER: Yes, you could do that. What else could you do?

By repetitive use of techniques such as this, the youth has an opportunity to practice the skills needed to address deficiencies in response generation. The technique can be expanded to allow the trainer to focus on the consequences of the proposed solutions. For example:

TRAINER: Let's say another student comes by and shuts your locker while you are looking for a book. What could you do?

YOUTH: I could smack him upside his head!

TRAINER: Yes, you could do that. What would most likely happen then?

YOUTH: We'd be goin' at it!

TRAINER: And what would be the consequence of that?

YOUTH: Probably get suspended.

TRAINER: Okay, what is another possible solution?

Interventions associated with deficiencies in Step 6 of the social-information-processing model, behavioral enactment of the selected response, will focus on behavioral skills training. There is a significant practical difference between simply "knowing about" nonaggressive responses and actually having the skills and motivation to enact them in authentic situations with the appropriate timing. For instance, in a provocative situation a youth may *know* that being verbally assertive will have more desirable consequences than physical aggression. However, he or she cannot and will not select verbal assertion if the requisite skills are lacking (Pepler, King, & Byrd, 1991). This is a serious and difficult training challenge and, unfortunately, perhaps the one most underaddressed by otherwise well-meaning practitioners. Training must utilize *in vitro* and *in vivo* exercises to expose youths to problematic situations in which they can practice the skills necessary for a nonaggressive response repetitively and with trainer feedback.

SUMMARY

Middle and high school students whose personal histories have been characterized by fighting and other forms of aggressive conflict resolution will not go easily into that good night of behavioral change. Aggression has been demonstrated to be very stable over time (e.g., Huesmann & Moise, 1998; Olweus, 1979) and particularly resistant to change as children age into young adulthood (Eron & Slaby, 1994; Larson, 1994). Simplistic "solutions" such as "get-tough," zero-tolerance disciplinary policies, in addition to disproportionately targeting minority students and contributing to school dropout, have not been shown to be effective in changing student behavior or improving school safety (see Peterson, Larson, & Skiba, 2001, for a review). Although clearly stated behavioral policies for students are essential to address the kinds of complex interpersonal dynamics that occasion student aggression, they are wholly insufficient in isolation. In similar fashion, therapist-led small-group skills training in anger and aggression management or classroom activities that stimulate discussion and reflection about aggressive beliefs or values are equally inadequate by themselves.

What is needed in order to have even a reasonable likelihood of assisting historically aggressive youths to learn the skills and benefits of nonviolent conflict resolution is an ecological approach that reaches into multiple domains of school life. The systems of administrative policy and decision making, classroom education, and school mental health service delivery must interact in a mutually supportive, prevention-oriented approach that focuses primarily on training nonviolent interpersonal skills in the school setting. How such an approach may be implemented is the subject of the remainder of this book.

CHAPTER 2

◆◆◆

The Context
of Aggressive Student Behavior

Creating Effective,
Whole-School Environmental Strategies

◆

In the course of my 14 years of experience as a school psychologist in a major urban school district and now as a university supervisor of interns and practicum students in a wide variety of school districts across my state, I have witnessed nearly the full spectrum of schoolwide order and disorder. My first assignment as a newly licensed school psychologist back in the mid-1970s was in an aging central city high school. The building was scheduled to be closed as a neighborhood high school and reopened the following year as a magnet school for college-bound students from across the city. This was to be its last academic year as a regular attendance area school for neighborhood families. During that final year, I witnessed a student body subjected to unapologetic lack of interest from the central administration and the predictable consequences for the teaching and learning environment that ensued. Students and nonstudents alike wandered the hallways during class time, ignoring or challenging any adult who attempted to intervene. Dice games went on in back corners, and fights were everywhere at all hours of the school day. Gang members openly displayed their colors, and adults in garish clothes and equally garish cars patrolled the front of the building awaiting the dismissal bell. What administrative "discipline" there was took the form of unrelenting suspensions and expulsions. The majority of the students, decent and desirous of an education, were left mostly to their own devices to limp safely through the school year. Some graduated; most of the rest were reassigned to other schools across the city.

That year was far and away the worst situation I ever observed. I went on to involvement in numerous other middle and high schools as a staff school psychologist and later as a consultant on the school system's Violence Reduction Program. These experiences have convinced me of two rather unstartling insights:

1. *Safe and effective learning environments arise out of the vision and efforts of strong leadership.* Like any well-managed corporation, a school building reflects the skills, drive, and competence of its leadership. Principals are in critically powerful positions to direct the learning and social climate of their buildings in a positive direction regardless of who spills into their hallways from the streets outside.

2. *Schools that care best about any group of students care equally about all groups of students.* The social-behavioral needs of the most competent students are inexorably tied to those of the least competent. The students in the in-school suspension room and the students in the advanced chemistry lab have a shared relationship with one another, whether they ever meet face-to-face as individuals or not. The most effective schools understand that and address the needs of both systematically, equally, and with evidence-based procedures.

The remainder of this chapter will address how the leadership element in a middle or high school can provide the kind of whole-school learning environment that reduces the likelihood of violent student interactions and simultaneously facilitates a climate most conducive to academic excellence and personal growth for all of the students. Let's begin by answering the question "Who's in charge here?"

LEADERSHIP

There are enormous pressures from parents and the general public for schools to be perceived as safe and effective. The reactive climate of fear and hypervigilance promulgated by the spate of school shootings that closed out the last millennium continues to hold considerable sway, and national polls show parents still very concerned about the safety of their children. A recent Gallup/Phi Delta Kappa poll (Rose & Gallup, 2003) found "lack of discipline and the need for more control" sharing the top of the list of public concerns with economic issues and "fighting, violence, and gangs" occupying the second slot. Many parents are still fearful about the possibility of school shootings occurring in their communities (Gallup Organization, 2001). The popularity of movies that show principals carrying baseball bats is testimony to the fear and frustration in many communities. It is therefore understandable that many schools have chosen to enact get-tough policies in an effort to weed out the troublemakers.

Strong leadership, however, means considerably more than establishing simplistic get-tough policies. One of my responsibilities as a professor in a school psychology training program is to make regular site visits to schools where my interns are placed. Recently, I was sitting in the principal's office of a large middle school discussing the progress of my intern when our conversation was interrupted by a loud commotion from the outer office. The principal excused himself and disappeared out the door to investigate. Moments later he returned, followed by two male students snarling under their breaths and elbowing one another. They remained standing in the center of the office. The principal informed me that the two had been escorted down by their teacher for fighting in the shop area. He then began what seemed to be a well-worn interrogation that went something like this:

PRINCIPAL: Tell me what happened.

STUDENTS: [Explanation]

PRINCIPAL: Why did you do that?

STUDENTS: [Explanation]

PRINCIPAL: What are the consequences for fighting in school?

STUDENTS: [Silence]

PRINCIPAL: Call your parents. You are both suspended for three days.

After an aide appeared to escort the two boys to their lockers, the principal told me that his predecessor had retired early, in part because of unremitting parental complaints about the behavior of the students in this building. Reestablishing order was his first priority, and "zero tolerance for fighting and disrespect to teachers" was the centerpiece of this effort. When I inquired about how things were going, he responded by informing me that whereas his predecessor was besieged with phone calls from the angry parents of well-behaved students who were being victimized, his calls were almost always from the angry parents of problem students whom he had suspended. His goal, he said, was to eventually eliminate most of those calls as well.

"Zero tolerance" is a term used to describe policies that establish predetermined consequences for various student offenses, such as violence, weapon carrying, and substance possession or use. "From its inception in federal drug policy of the 1980s, zero tolerance has been intended primarily as a method of sending a message that certain behaviors will not be tolerated, by punishing all offenses severely, no matter how minor" (Skiba, 2000, p. 2). Zero tolerance is one of those no-nonsense, get-tough, shape-up-or-ship-out expressions loved by all those in the general public who believe that the inmates are in charge down at the old junior high. The presumed logic is that one need only have zero tolerance for something bad and it will disappear. In this respect, "zero tolerance" is the educational equivalent of "just say no."

In fairness, the concept of zero tolerance seems to have some highly targeted usefulness in the education of children. The federal government, in its 1994 Safe and Gun Free Schools Act, mandated that states enact laws declaring that any student caught with a firearm in or within 1,000 feet of a school building must be remanded to the criminal courts and expelled from school for at least 1 year. Addressing the weapons problem in schools is clearly a serious concern. The Centers for Disease Control and Prevention (CDC, 2003) reported that in 2001, 17.4% of U.S. high school students had carried a weapon—gun, knife, or club—in the 30 days prior to the survey, with 5.7% carrying a gun and 6.4% carrying a weapon on school property. The notion of "zero tolerance" for such behavior is both understandable and, to some degree, enforceable. Indeed, trend data over the past decade has shown a modest decline in weapon carrying in schools (CDC, 2003). Anecdotes about expelled first graders with squirt guns aside, getting tough with weapons on campus has been generally well received in the educational community.

Applying a zero-tolerance-style disciplinary approach to more typical school problems, however, does not yield similar results. In their review of the zero-tolerance research, Skiba and Peterson (1999) found "virtually no data to suggest that zero-tolerance policies reduce school violence" (p. 376). They went on to conclude: "Ultimately, as we commit ourselves to increasingly draconian policies of school discipline, we may also need to resign ourselves to increasingly joyless schools, increasingly unsafe streets, and dramatically increasing expenditures for detention centers and prisons" (p. 381).

The great majority of administrators are well aware that simply publishing a list of banned student behaviors is futile, particularly as an attempt to make an impact on the most grievous offenders. Try to imagine this occurring in the mind of a student with aggressive problem behavior:

> "Say, I think he bumped into me on purpose! I'd really like to haul off and smack him one, but the school now has a zero tolerance for fighting rule and if I did, I might get suspended and have to stay home and play video games for three days! Instead, I think I'll just continue on to class."

Not a very likely scenario, in my experience. Strong leadership in response to addressing the problem of interpersonal violence among students involves much more than establishing "tough rules."

Strong leadership does not require a commanding, charismatic personality; these qualities hardly describe Bill Gates or, for that matter, most of the strongest principals I have known. From my experience with principals over the years, I am convinced that leadership can be behavioralized: It is a matter of doing what effective leaders do. Administrators skilled in leadership understand that in order to create any form of effective and lasting change in their buildings, they must do the following: (1) help create the vision for change, (2) empower all the potential change agents, and (3) support and monitor the change as it occurs. This is no less true for the creation of a school environment of nonviolence than it is for any other major educational initiative.

CREATING THE VISION FOR CHANGE

In his excellent book, *Visionary Leadership*, Nanus (1992) wrote, "There is no more powerful engine driving an organization toward excellence and long-range success than an attractive, worthwhile and achievable vision of the future, widely shared" (p. 3). When a principal decides to address the level of violence in his or her learning environment, the first task of leadership is to create a vision for change, or, as Covey (1992) suggested, "Begin with the end in mind" (p. 270). The initial impetus may originate with a single individual—a principal, a teacher, or a parent—but the vision, the knowledge of what the change will bring, must come from everyone affected. As Oakley and Krug (1991) observed:

> Enlightened leaders actually don't need to have the vision themselves; they need only possess the willingness and the ability to draw the vision from their people and inspire and empower those people to do what it takes to bring the vision into reality. (p. 19)

A vision is a statement of direction, not a prophecy for the future. It describes what lies at the end of the journey but does not detail the path. A good vision statement reflects high ideals, clarifies direction, inspires enthusiasm, and demonstrates ambition for greater achievements (Nanus, 1991). Vision statements move beyond traditional school mission statements to actually *imagine what the school will be like.* Consider this example:

> "We envision a school where all students, staff, and visitors interact with civility, mutual respect, and compassion. Disagreements are resolved without verbal threat or physical aggression. We envision a school wherein systems and programs are in place to meet the knowledge and skill development of all students, including and particularly those who must struggle to maintain this vision. Our discipline is educational, not purely punitive, and strives to provide the student with knowledge and skill to avoid future difficulties of a similar kind. Our vision is inclusive of diversity in all its forms, including racial, ethnic, learning, and behavioral."

The first order of business for the principal is to bring together a representative group of the most energetic, thoughtful, and positive-thinking individuals in the building and create that vision. The mechanism for coming together to create this critical initial document may already exist in many schools. Collaborative decision making in the form of school leadership teams, site-based management teams, parent advisory councils, and individualized education programming teams has become a fixture in most school districts in the 21st century. School people are used to addressing problems in a collaborative manner; consequently, in many schools there may already be an existing vehicle for developing the vision. The goal is to make the vision reflective of the school community as a whole, not merely that of a single visionary or interest group, so representative participation is essential. Teachers, students, parents, community members—including law enforcement—and noninstructional staff all have stakes in the vision, and all should be a part of the creative process. The brainstorming activity described in Figure 2.1 can be a useful place to begin.

Once the vision statement is complete, the time has come to share it with the greater school community. It is critical that this not be an afterthought but, rather, built in at the onset and viewed as an essential aspect of what will eventually bring the vision to fruition. Every communication outlet should be considered, both those internal to the school and those that reach the citizens in the community. In many circumstances, school leadership will find it necessary to "sell" this new vision to what may be skeptical or even openly hostile audiences. High levels of entrenched negativity and pessimism in some buildings and communities will present a chal-

---

Opening activity: Brainstorming the vision

Tack a sheet of butcher paper to the wall. Provide each member with a package of sticky-note pads. On separate individual sticky notes, instruct each member to write responses to:

"If there was no more violence or threat of violence in our school,
what changes would we see?"

- Limit responses to one per sticky note.
- Encourage as many responses as possible, allowing members to address changes in whatever or whomever they choose.
- Encourage ambitious, even improbable responses. This is a brainstorming activity, so there are no constraints on the imagination!
- Have members paste their responses on the butcher paper anywhere.
- When everyone has finished sticking their notes on the paper, have them all gather at the butcher paper and move the sticky notes into logical groupings and label them.
- Typical groupings in this activity are changes in: students, teachers, administrators, parents, physical environment, general and classroom climate, budgetary expenditures, and disciplinary procedures.

What is now on the butcher paper is the unedited first form of the vision statement. The role of the group at this juncture is to put the suggestions into priority and create generalized wording that reflects the agreed-upon priorities. Remember that the vision statement is meant to *inspire* change, not detail its every manifestation.

FIGURE 2.1. A vision of nonviolence worksheet.

lenge. For some educators to have a "here we go again!" attitude is quite understand-able. One does not have to work in a school district very long to watch one "impor-tant initiative" after another come along, only to be forgotten or replaced in quick order. It is important that leadership remain openly committed to the vision in word and deed, keep it on the agenda, and persevere in the process to carry it out.

Readers who want to examine further the issues of facilitating the creation of visions and processes for change may consult any of the following: Garmston and Wellman (1999), Hall and Hord (1987), Knoff (2002), Nanus (1992), and Senge et al. (2000).

VISION INTO REALITY: A THREE-TIERED APPROACH

What then is the most effective course of action for school administrators to take in their efforts to curb interpersonal student violence and instill an environment most conducive to learning for all of the students? This is where "strong leadership" meets "caring for all students." Principals have substantial influence over the "setting events" of their buildings. That is, they have the power to exert influence over the environmental and social conditions that can increase or decrease the likelihood of problem behavior. When administrators approach this issue in a considered and sys-tematic fashion, they consider the requirements of all the students for a disciplinary structure that addresses each individual's level of need for external assistance.

A useful and increasingly well-supported methodology for creating a school environment that meets the behavioral needs of all students conceptualizes student disciplinary needs in a three-tiered pyramid (Figure 2.2) that follows a public health prevention model (Furlong, Morrison, Austin, Huh-Kim, & Skager, 2001; Larson, Smith, & Furlong, 2002; Walker et al., 1996). Approximately 60–70% of the typical school population are at the base of the pyramid. These are students for whom *pri-mary prevention* planning is sufficient. Students in this category generally have com-paratively higher levels of self-discipline and behavior management skills than some of their peers. Programs and procedures within a primary prevention focus are referred to as "universal prevention programs." Further up the pyramid is a smaller subset of the student population consisting of those students who, because of per-sonal characteristics or environmental factors, are at serious risk for continuing aca-demic and behavioral problems. Disciplinary programs designed to meet the needs of these individuals are known as *secondary* prevention, and the procedures used are referred to as *selected prevention measures*. Last, at the top of the pyramid and mak-ing up the smallest group of students, are individuals with the greatest needs for external disciplinary programs and supports. *Tertiary prevention* services are designed to address the needs of these students, whose behavior has been unrespon-sive to universal or selected prevention procedures. These programs are referred to as "indicated prevention measures."

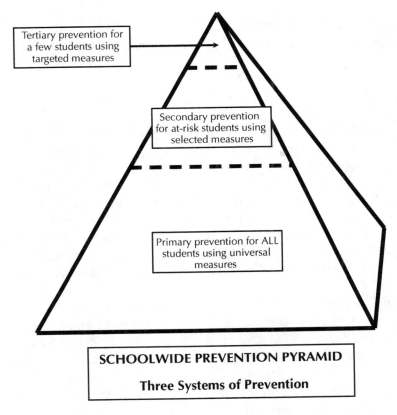

Tertiary prevention for a few students using targeted measures

Secondary prevention for at-risk students using selected measures

Primary prevention for ALL students using universal measures

SCHOOLWIDE PREVENTION PYRAMID

Three Systems of Prevention

FIGURE 2.2. Three-tiered prevention pyramid.

Universal Prevention Programs

The majority of students in a typical middle or high school come to school with the requisite skills and dispositions to engage effectively and with few problems in the learning experience. In general, these students require only knowledge and understanding of the school or classroom rules and conduct expectations in order to enact their existing skills and dispositions to adhere to them. Because they often contrast so favorably with their more problematic peers, adults frequently neglect the fact that these students also have prevention needs in the area of behavioral discipline. These needs are best met in effective schoolwide codes of conduct and individual classroom rules.

Codes and rules are antecedent-based behavior management programs in that they are designed to prevent the enactment of problem behavior by manipulating the setting events to reinforce predetermined desired behaviors. Well-designed codes and classroom rules assist the students in their efforts to engage in behavior that will be reinforced and avoid behavior that will not. Knowledge of a code principle or a particular classroom rule does not, of itself, cause students to alter their behavior, but it increases the likelihood that many will. Let us examine these two primary prevention programs.

Codes of Conduct

A code of conduct is a vital aspect of an overall school discipline plan in that it helps establish a norm of expected behavior and serves to justify actions needed to address problem behavior among the students (O'Donnell, 2001). Through its official sanction by a governing school board, a code of conduct brings the behavioral expectations of the local community into the schoolhouse. Shannon and McCall (2003), in their review of North American school discipline codes, concluded "that school policies that set reasonable, clearly understood, actively enforced behavioural expectations for students and staff can be effective in protecting the safety of all students as well as in correcting the behaviours of offending students" (Behavioural Expectations section, para. 5).

Creating an effective code of conduct is more than merely drawing up a list of undesirable behaviors and connecting them to some form of aversive consequence, however. Too often, codes are devised by the adults in the system and distributed to the students in a manner more akin to a threat than a learning experience. An effective code does not float menacingly above the student body like some dark angel ready to enact vengeance upon the transgressor for stepping out of line. Rather, a meaningful code of conduct is organic to the system; it permeates every interaction and helps define the nature of the learning environment. When the code of conduct is essentially indistinguishable from the other learning and social activities within which it is embedded, then its potential for effectiveness is maximized.

As an example, when emotionally healthy adults come together for a social gathering, there is a "code of conduct" that is embedded in the event that purposefully, but imperceptibly, allows the goals of the event to be met. There is nothing written. No one is handed a card with "do's and don'ts" as they arrive. The "code" is there, rooted in the learned behavior of the participants, and emerges into consciousness only in the event of its breach. The likelihood of such a gathering being pleasant and satisfying to the participants is related in large part to the maturity of the participants and the fact that everyone is gathered for pretty much the same purpose.

In contrast, middle and high schools are social environments at which multiple individuals with diverse levels of maturity arrive each morning with goals that, in some circumstances, are in direct conflict with the goals of others.

"I'm here to learn."
"I'm here to have as much fun as I possibly can."
"I'm here to teach."
"I'm here just to avoid a truancy bust."
"I'm here to help my teachers do their jobs."

"I'm here to sell drugs."

"I'm here to protect my pension."

And so on. If it were as simple as "all of the students are here to learn, and all of the teachers are here to teach," then manufacturing a written code to guide behavior would be unnecessary. Alas . . .

Codes of conduct generally originate as broadly worded state statutes that establish mandates and guidelines for local school boards to follow (Redding & Shalf, 2001). For instance, in the state of Wisconsin, the following statutory wording guides the local districts:

> **120.13 School board powers.** The school board of a common or union high school district may do all things reasonable to promote the cause of education, including establishing, providing and improving school district programs, functions and activities for the benefit of pupils, and including all of the following:
>
> (1) SCHOOL GOVERNMENT RULES; SUSPENSION; EXPULSION. (a) Make rules for the organization, gradation and government of the schools of the school district, including rules pertaining to conduct and dress of pupils in order to maintain good decorum and a favorable academic atmosphere, which shall take effect when approved by a majority of the school board and filed with the school district clerk. (Wisconsin State Statutes, 120.13[1][a]).

Local school boards receive legislative mandates such as these and create district policy. As an example, in response to the legislative mandate, the Madison Metropolitan School District (2003) in Wisconsin created a districtwide Code of Conduct that governs all individuals in the district. The code addresses the following major categories:

I. Classroom Code of Conduct
   A. Rights and Responsibilities of Student and Parents
   B. Rights and Responsibilities of Teachers
   C. Rights and Responsibilities of Administrators
   D. Definitions
II. Student Conduct and Discipline Plan
   A. Student and Parent Rights
   B. Student Responsibilities
   C. Parent Responsibilities
III. District Suspension Codes
   A. Conduct which Impeded the Orderly Operation of the Classroom or School
   B. Illegal or Serious Misconduct—Not Life or Health Threatening
   C. Serious and/or Illegal Misconduct—Life, Health Threatening, or Repeated Conduct that Disrupts the Educational Process

The developmental process and content of useful and effective codes of conduct have been discussed in reviews (e.g., Day, Golench, MacDougall, & Beals-Gonzalez, 1995; Gottfredson, 1997; Redding & Shalf, 2001; Shannon & McCall, 2003) and in policy statements (e.g., U.S. Department of Education, 1998). In addition, Redding and Shaft provided Internet addresses of 11 exemplar codes of conduct from across the United States. Drawing on these resources, the following elements of an effective code of conduct are offered:

1. *The code should arise legitimately out of official School Board business.* As Shannon and McCall (2003) noted, it is important for codes to have legitimacy within the system and to reflect the will of the elected representatives of the community of who sit on the school board. The impetus for the code and the finalized document itself must have a record in the recognized policy-making procedures of the school board. In this sense, the code obtains a degree of legal status for disciplinary due process matters in the school.

2. *The code should be developed in a collaborative manner.* Whether a school is rewriting an existing code of conduct or starting from scratch, input and ownership from all major stakeholders is essential. If the code is to be an integral part of the school's prevention program, then it must be informed by those most closely associated with its implementation. Along with building administrators, representation on the code-writing team should include: teachers (general and special education), students, supportive services staff (guidance, school psychology, school social work), parents, school security, and community law enforcement. Each interest group should be asked to address concerns relative to its area of expertise. For example:

- *Teachers*: What elements in a code are essential to the maintenance of an environment most conducive to teaching and learning in the classroom? How can the code be written so that most students and parents can understand its meaning and intent? What separate adaptations in wording or form are needed so that students and parents with special needs are provided with equal opportunity to understand the code? How can the code be reorganized into a teachable curriculum? What are the most effective and reasonable procedures for teaching the code (e.g., integration into classroom content, special modules, assemblies, and so on)?
- *Students*: What are the positive behaviors in peers and adults in the school setting that students want to see encouraged by the code? What are the negative behaviors that should be deterred or punished by the code? What interpersonal problems among the students are distinctive to this school and should be addressed in the code (e.g., gang issues, student cliques or societies, racial issues, sexual harassment, and so on)? What word usage in the code is out of date or confusing and should be replaced?

- *Supportive services*: How can the code be constructed to promote optimum mental health for all individuals in the school setting? How does research on the developmental needs and characteristics of adolescents inform the content of the code? How can the code be integrated most effectively with the counseling and intervention skills and schedules of the supportive services staff members? What are the prevention needs of the most behaviorally at-risk students that should be addressed in the code?
- *Law enforcement*: What behaviors designated in the code are also violations of the criminal or juvenile statutes and need to be brought to the attention of law enforcement?

3. *The code should reflect the singular setting, mission, and participants of the school.* As far as school codes of conduct go, there is no "one size fits all." Although any school can learn from the code of another school—and consulting other codes is prudent—ultimately the school's code must reflect the uniqueness of its own students and goals. Obtaining this individuality comes from a clear vision of the needs of the students and the purpose for which they attend *this* particular school. Continuous mention of the school's name throughout the document (e.g., "Students at Washington High School understand that. . . . ") will help both the writers and the readers focus on the issues and persons germane to the school in consideration. An excellent example of a code uniquely composed for a specific population may be found at the website for the Pegasus Charter School in Dallas, Texas (*www.pegasuscharter.org*). This school is located in central Dallas and serves a population of racially and economically diverse students in grades 7–12.

4. *The code should clearly articulate its role and purpose in the lives of the affected individuals.* The creation of an introductory purpose statement should be one of the first tasks of the code-writing team. Initially for the writers and later for the readers, the purpose statement describes the reasons that such a code is necessary and defines its relationship to the mission of the school. Creating this purpose at the onset of the code-writing effort will assist the writers to maintain their focus on the agreed-upon function of the code and deter the urge to overburden the document with material that arguably belongs elsewhere. At a minimum, the purpose statement should include the answers to the following:

- What is the mission of the school, briefly stated?
- In what ways does this code of conduct assist in that mission?
- Who are the individuals whose conduct will be guided by this code?

5. *The code should address the conduct of everyone involved in the school, not just the students.* The document should be titled a "Code of Conduct for _____ School," not a "Student Code of Conduct," and should address rights, responsibilities, and conduct for everyone involved in the educational process.

Secondary-level students are much attuned to "fairness," and a document handed down from the adults addressing exclusively what students should and should not do may be less well received than a more globally oriented code. "Student conduct codes" convey an "us against them" tone that is antithetical to the goal of a code to establish a norm of behavior in the building. Not only is it important for students to see that the adults have expected norms just as they do, but also codifying educator and parent normative expectations can be useful in new employee training and any potential due process proceedings that may subsequently occur. Examples of articulated student, parent, and staff rights and responsibilities may be found at the Madison (Wisconsin) Metropolitan School District website (*www.madison.k12.wi.us/policies/4502.htm*) and the Arlington (Texas) Independent School District website (*www.arlington.k12.tx.us/pdf/coc.pdf*).

6. *The code should clearly communicate and encourage responsibility and desirable behaviors.* The document should be a teaching tool for success that assists in everyone's decision-making process. An effective code of conduct goes well beyond the mere enumeration of prohibited behaviors. More than just a statement of rules and disciplinary procedures, an effective code also details the kinds of dispositions and behaviors that will lead to success within the environment. The question for the code-writing team is, What are the behaviors and attitudes we want in our students, staff, and parents? In essence the code should articulate just what the members of the school community should be doing when they conduct themselves in a manner most conducive to pursuing the mission of the school. These elements should be carefully considered by the code-writing team and written in positive phrasing. For example, the Arlington (Texas) Independent School District (*www.arlington.k12.tx.us/pdf/coc.pdf*) encourages students to "Express opinions and ideas in a respectful manner," "Cooperate with all lawful and reasonable directives issued by school personnel," and "Strive toward self-discipline, setting individual goals, and utilizing good work habits" (Arlington Independent School District, 2003; Student Responsibilities section).

7. *The code should clearly articulate student and staff member rights.* A code of school conduct cannot abridge rights guaranteed to students and staff by federal or state authority. An effective code articulates those rights most germane to the school setting in developmentally appropriate language and provides examples for student understanding. The Montgomery County (Maryland) Public Schools (*www.mcps.k12.md.us/departments/publishingservices/PDF/studntrr.pdf*) and the Fairfax (Virginia) County Public Schools (*www.fcps.k12.va.us*) have comprehensive and well-written sections that detail student and adult rights as they pertain to the school setting.

8. *The code should clearly articulate, define, and provide examples of those actions and behaviors that are prohibited.* One of the essential functions of a code of conduct is to place reasonable boundaries on the behavior of those persons under its auspices. Clarity and specificity in this section are paramount.

- Identify the behavior in observable terms. Avoid terminology such as "disruptive behavior" or "aggressive behavior" without substantial additional clarification and a list of the most frequently observed examples.
- Identify the physical locations that are under the auspices of the code. Are these behaviors also prohibited on the bus? On the walk to and from school? In the community during field trips?
- Identify the times that the code is in effect. Under what circumstances are these behaviors prohibited during nonschool hours? For instance, in an infamous Northbrook, Illinois, powder puff football game hazing incident, the school needed to decide whether its code prohibitions against hazing obtained on the weekend in a nonsanctioned event.
- Identify the legal authority behind the prohibition. Is the behavior, class of behaviors, or prohibitory action identified in existing school board regulations? Is the behavior identified in the state juvenile, criminal, or civil rights codes?

9. *The code should include distinctions between minor and serious violations.* Prohibited behaviors that the code is designed to deter should be identified on a continuum of severity. The overwhelming majority of code violations are minor infractions (failure to bring supplies, tardiness, swearing, and other acts of minor misconduct), but their inclusion in the code is essential from a "quality of educational life" standpoint. These less serious violations are the first veneer on the normative floor. Their identification and successful disciplinary response can have an effect on the frequency of "next level" violations. For these behaviors, the code should encourage less formal, classroom-level responses, increasing from low intensity, primarily corrective actions to mild punishment. Following this continuum approach, the code should go on to identify increasingly serious groupings of behaviors and link them to a rationally conceived range of disciplinary responses. The Arlington (Texas) Independent School District (*arlington.k12.tx.us/pdf/coc.pdf*) and the Leon County (Florida) School District (*www.planning.leon.k12.fl.us/Policies/708.htm*) have developed examples of this type of code construction.

10. *The code should be preventive and educational and include procedures to assist individuals who violate it.* The code-writing team should be ever cognizant of the educational mission of public schools and should reflect that awareness throughout the code of conduct. Not only should the code articulate and encourage appropriate behavior, but it should also have parallel goals of preventing and remediating inappropriate behavior. It does no good to send a behaviorally unskilled student to school or home detention and anticipate that he or she will somehow magically acquire the skills necessary to avoid a subsequent violation. Disciplinary responses in each category of infraction should include a mandatory, evidence-supported educational or skill development component individualized to the unique needs of the student. The goal of such a component is to reduce the likelihood that the student will

subsequently select the prohibited behavior in similar circumstances by providing the knowledge or skills necessary for an alternative response.

11. *The code should be taught to all students in a manner consistent with effective instructional practices.* The practice of merely distributing a copy of the code of conduct and instructing students that they are now responsible for its contents must be abandoned. Regardless of any stern warnings on the cover sheet (or even the effort to require parent signatures), information treated in this manner comes with the implied message that it is not a learning priority for the student or a teaching priority for the staff. Complex information distributed only as a reading assignment is poor pedagogy regardless of the subject matter, and holding students subsequently responsible for its content is educationally indefensible. Ninth-grade English and math are important educational priorities, and this is evidenced by the time, effort, and creativity that most often accompany the curricula. Helping students to understand the complexities of the code of conduct in a similar manner communicates its importance and increases the likelihood that the code will have its intended influence. Targeting the incoming class of students with a few minutes set aside each day at the onset of the year can potentially "pay for itself" with reduced disciplinary concerns in the months to come. The following is a suggested procedure:

- Render all sections of the code to a series of teaching modules and learner outcomes. Identify what the students will "know and be able to do" at the conclusion of each module, and create appropriate assessment procedures.
- Facilitate the opportunity for master teachers to convert the learner outcomes into effective, teacher-friendly pedagogical procedures and activities, with an eye toward minimizing classroom teacher preparation time in order to teach it.
- Identify the most logical and reasonable classes or opportunities (e.g., homeroom) for the curriculum to be taught, and train those instructors in the curriculum.
- Implement the curriculum with all of the students in the first year and target the incoming students in the years to come, with refresher lessons for older students.
- Consider training a group of students as a "traveling role-play troupe" to visit each classroom and provide live examples of critical or confusing aspects of the code.

12. *The code should be revisited on a yearly basis for updates and refinements.* After the school shootings that occurred in the late 1990s, many school codes of conduct were changed to reflect what was perceived as the new reality for heightened security and school safety. In a similar fashion, increasing use of computers in the school setting has brought on the need for limit setting and guidance for their use. Administrators should include code updating as a regular item in the year's end

agenda of their school policymaking structure so as to have the newest iteration available for the start of the new school year.

As a further resource, educators Stein, Richin, Banyon, Banyon, and Stein (2000) have written a unique and practical book, *Connecting Character to Conduct: Helping Students Do the Right Things*, in which they expand on what they see as four critical principles of student conduct: respect, impulse control, compassion, and equity. These principles are translated into student behavior standards across multiple school settings, and, using the imaginary school district of "Centerville," the authors describe how the principles can be integrated and taught within the existing curriculum.

Just as the code of conduct helps to define the nature of the overall learning environment of the school, classroom rules apply similar principles to the idiosyncratic needs of individual curricular environments. Classroom rules are an essential universal prevention measure that allows the code to be individualized to meet specific environmental needs where "the rubber meets the road" in the schooling process.

Classroom Rules

A teacher friend of mine used to joke that he began each year by showing his students his "Two Simple Rules for Success in My Classroom":

Rule 1: Do what I tell you to do.
Rule 2: See Rule 1.

Levity aside, the establishment of a short list of rules to guide student behavior in the classroom is one the most important aspects of a primary prevention program. Classroom rules may be seen as individualizing the code of conduct to the unique circumstances of a particular classroom and establishing a norm of behavior for that environment. Rules for the chemistry lab, the locker room, or the English classroom will differ qualitatively, but they should all be intended to encourage the kinds of responsible, self-disciplined behaviors identified in the code of conduct.

Similar to the broader school code, classroom rules exert their influence at the antecedent or prevention level, affecting the choice of behavior before it is enacted. A student enters a classroom and immediately seeks to engage in behaviors that he or she believes will obtain reinforcement or avoid discomfort. Some may immediately take their seats and ready themselves for the lesson, others may chat with friends, and still others may engage in horseplay. The students all select behaviors that they believe to be in their best interest, based on their individual set of knowledge, skills, and experience. Their common goals are to (1) continue or begin a reinforcing condition, or (2) discontinue or avoid an aversive one.

For example, Jennifer knows that she can continue her conversation with Sara, a reinforcing condition, until the teacher finally shouts at her to sit down. At that time, she knows she can avoid the aversive condition of an office referral by complying. Juan knows that if he readies himself for the lecture as soon as he gets to the room, he can avoid the aversive condition of trying to play catch-up with the material for the whole class. James knows that if he continues his horseplay behavior, the teacher will send him out, relieving him of the aversive condition of a class he does not enjoy. Seek pleasure, avoid pain: It's what we humans do.

In effect, well-written classroom rules provide information as to which behaviors will be reinforced by the teacher in that particular setting. For that large majority of typically unproblematic students, that information is generally sufficient. Provided with such behavioral guidelines, that group is able to select behaviors that will define the expected norms for that classroom. In other words, well-written classroom rules help the students who want to and are able to engage in academically desirable behaviors to do just that. When that group is demonstrating those behaviors, they have the potential to be a powerful model for their less skilled or less motivated peers. Absent reasonable and consistently enforced rules, even the least historically problematic students may seek reinforcement from other sources (e.g., peers) or begin to avoid the environment entirely.

Walker, Colvin, and Ramsey (1995) advised that classroom rules should be (1) explicitly stated, (2) functional, (3) established on the first day of class, (4) rehearsed, and (4) practiced. Rules should be clear enough so that there is little or no room for interpretation on anyone's part. One should strictly avoid inexplicit words such as "respect," "inappropriate," or "unacceptable," as they lend themselves easily to personal judgment. Instead, phrase the rules in positive, functional terms that communicate what the teacher wants the students to do. Walker et al. (1995, p. 157) offered 11 sample rule phrasings, including the following:

- Be on time for class.
- Enter the classroom quietly.
- Go to your assigned areas promptly.
- Listen to the teacher's directions or explanations.
- Raise your hand if you wish to talk or need assistance.

Notice that the rules instruct the students in the desired behaviors and that each is conducive to the maintenance of a positive learning environment. Keeping the list to between three and six will facilitate easier assimilation and accommodation (Striepling, 1997).

The first day of class is the most advantageous time to establish rules in the classroom, as it negates the need for both the teacher and the class to have to possibly unlearn bad habits. With adolescents, including them as collaborators in the effort to establish rules is a developmentally important element (Hyman, 1997). Rather than simply announcing the rules, teachers will find that devoting the first 20–30 minutes of Day 1 to working with the students on "our classroom rules" will be beneficial. The teacher should know ahead of time the areas that he or she wants addressed with positive, functional rules and guide the classroom discussion accordingly. For example:

> "This classroom is like a workplace environment. Your job is to learn [the curriculum], and my job is to help you do that. In order for each of us to do our jobs effectively and minimize problems, we have to agree on some rules for getting along together. My experience is that rules are best stated in terms of what you are supposed to do, rather than what you aren't supposed to do. For instance, a rule in a mechanic's shop might say, 'Return tools to their proper place when finished,' rather than 'Don't leave tools lying around.' This way, the workers know exactly what is expected. Let's start by thinking about entering into our classroom from the hallway at the beginning of class. Let me see raised hands with suggestions about a rule that will help us avoid problems during that transition. How should everyone enter the classroom?"

Exact phrasing of the rules can be left to the teacher for later rendering to a large poster (see, e.g. Figure 2.3), but the critical feature is that the students see themselves as collaborators in the process, that they feel a genuine sense of ownership. Teachers should remember, however, that the students are collaborating with them, not dictating to them: Never include a rule that runs counter to a safe, orderly learning environment or that cannot be applied fairly and consistently, and never leave out a rule that is personally important.

Once written, the rules must be taught. Five minutes at the beginning of each class for the first week and then a booster lesson or two as needed thereafter is generally sufficient. Teachers should use a discuss–model–rehearse procedure to clarify the intent of each rule. For instance, when a student has "all necessary supplies," what does that mean? Does "Proceed directly to your desk and be seated" mean that a student cannot stop to speak with the teacher? What is the difference between a "low-

- Take care of all necessary personal grooming before entering the classroom.
- Enter quietly and proceed directly to your assigned seat.
- Place only required supplies on the desktop.
- Speak in a low-volume voice until class is called to order, then be silent with head up and eyes forward.
- Raise your hand and be recognized before speaking.
- Remain in your seat until dismissed or receiving teacher permission.

FIGURE 2.3. Example classroom rules for lecture-based middle or high school classrooms.

volume voice" and a *not* "low-volume voice?" Teachers should have students demonstrate rule adherence and rule nonadherence for clarification purposes.

Now that the rules are established and taught, an important point to remember
is that *when a rule is broken, an aversive consequence must follow every time.* This
principle is what distinguishes a "rule" from any other guide or influence on classroom behavior. It is not a suggestion or preference for behavior; it is an agreed-upon
standard that cannot be breached without consequence. Fair and consistent enforcement of the rules, particularly early on, will help cement that principle in the minds
of the students and allow the rules to function as they were intended, that is, to set a
norm of acceptable behavior.

One caveat: If an otherwise rule-adhering student regularly violates a particular
rule in spite of the aversive consequences, the teacher should consider the likelihood
that a *skill deficit* rather than a *motivational deficit* exists ("Can't do" vs. "Won't
do"). Whereas most behaviorally unproblematic students have the ability to regulate
their conduct to conform to a rule, some students simply do not have the skill to do
so and require additional supports. A problem-solving conference with the student,
in addition to consultation with school supportive services personnel, may be necessary to define and enact necessary behavioral supports.

Universal prevention programs address the potential for aggressive student
behavior by establishing an environmental norm of nonviolence and predictable, civil
procedural order. The large majority of students who are characteristically disinclined to violence are provided behavioral guideposts and official support for their
nonaggressive behavior. In turn, the behavior of these students provides positive
models and helps to create innumerable setting events around the school that serve to
reduce the likelihood of problem behavior among their more aggressive peers.

Selected Prevention Procedures

Although universal prevention programs are essential components, they are by themselves insufficient to create a schoolwide environment that is free from interpersonal
aggression. School leaders must also take steps to address the needs of that subset of
students who lack either the skills or personal dispositions to respond to these prevention measures. Students with chronic patterns of disruptive, aggressive behavior
need more highly individualized support and more focused opportunities to acquire
the skills for behavioral success in school (Sugai, Sprague, Horner, & Walker, 2001;
Walker et al., 1996; Walker, Ramsey, & Gresham, 2004). These students are consequently *selected* for additional attention. When school personnel fail to provide adequate support and training and instead direct only punitive sanctions and their own
frustration at the misbehaving students, both parties lose.

The establishment of schoolwide environmental supports (also referred to as
positive behavioral supports [PBS], effective behavioral supports [EBS], or positive

behavioral interventions and supports [PBIS]) had its genesis in the special education inclusion movement (see Carr et al., 1999, for a review) and has recently been adopted for the needs of the general education population, including students with disruptive, aggressive behavior. "Positive behavioral support is a general term that refers to the application of positive behavioral interventions and systems to achieve socially important behavior change" (Sugai et al., 1999, p. 6). The work of George Sugai and his colleagues (e.g., Eber, Sugai, Smith, & Scott, 2002; Horner, Sugai, Lewis-Palmer, & Todd, 2001; Sugai & Horner, 1999; Sugai & Lewis, 1999) has provided a model for the implementation of environmental supports that addresses the needs of all students, including those with challenging behaviors.

Environmental supports are implemented on the three-tiered primary, secondary, and tertiary model described earlier. Effective schoolwide codes of conduct and skilled classroom management procedures anchor the first, primary prevention tier. At the second tier (secondary prevention), at-risk students who do not respond to the universal interventions are selected for additional supports and interventions. These selected prevention measures may take the form of behavioral skills training, academic support, adjusted school day, behavioral contracting, mentoring, or other research-supported interventions (Walker et al., 1996).

Although a well-designed, valid, and reliable screening and identification process is a critical component of selected prevention efforts at the early-elementary level (see Walker et al., 2004, for a useful model), it is a less complex undertaking at the middle and high school levels. Students with chronic disruptive or aggressive behavior problems, by and large, have "outed" themselves by the time they transition to middle or high school. Elementary school fifth graders with problem behavior become middle school sixth graders with problem behavior much more often than they undergo substantive behavioral change on their own over the intervening summer. This fact has critical implications for school officials at the lower level "feeder schools." These individuals should routinely provide the names of and summaries of prevention efforts with all high-risk students to the receiving school so that effective procedures may be continued and previous failures avoided. Special education programs are generally accomplished in this manner of transition planning, and general education officials can take an important lesson from them. Useful communication with the next level of schooling is certainly preferable to the implied belief in a "magic summer" of behavioral change.

Similar to the elementary level, a critical feature of selected procedures at the secondary level is obtaining well-designed assessment data that link the intervention to the individual needs of the student with problem behavior. A common barrier to effective behavioral support in many secondary schools is what is known as "one size fits all" thinking. In these occurrences, some form of "at-risk" program is administratively established, and all behaviorally and academically problematic students are shuffled in and out with little regard to their individual differences. This approach often takes the form of an isolated "at-risk room" staffed by an adult who at best offers mature counsel and academic support or at worst supervises a holding tank. Academic support or even wise counsel can be important in the school life of youths with high levels of anger-fueled aggression, but there is no research that indicates that either can provide the skills necessary for the students to avoid the problem. The additional downside for the students comes when they subsequently and predictably engage in aggressive behavior, and the school gives up on them or refers them to special education because they "have not responded to at-risk programming."

Effective interventions for behaviorally high-risk students must be informed by individual assessments that usefully define the behavior in terms of its function and the contextual environmental contingencies that encourage and maintain it. Functional behavioral assessment (FBA) is a procedure that can effectively gather the information necessary to design positive behavioral supports. In this process, the term "function" refers to "the purposes the behavior may serve in the environment" (Kazdin, 2001). The individual conducting the FBA on a student with aggressive behavior seeks information that will allow hypotheses to be generated regarding the purpose such aggression serves for the student. Does it serve the function of allowing the youth to escape from aversive interpersonal circumstances? Does it provide anger release? Does it bring peer approval? In addition, an FBA seeks to better define the environmental elements that both increase the likelihood of and serve as predictors for the behavior.

O'Neill et al. (1997, p. 3; emphasis in original) defined the five primary outcomes of a functional behavior assessment:

1. A clear *description of the problem behaviors*.
2. Identification of the events, times and situations that *predict* when the problem behavior *will* and *will not* occur across the full range of typical daily routines.
3. Identification of the *consequences that maintain the problem behaviors* (that is, what functions the behaviors appear to serve for the person).
4. Development of one or more *summary statements* or hypotheses that describe specific behaviors, a specific type of situation in which they occur, and the outcome reinforcers maintaining them in that situation.
5. Collection of *direct observation data* that support the summary statements that have been developed.

This information may be gathered directly through observation or indirectly through interview or behavioral checklists. A sample basic FBA interview form ("Current Behavior Screening Form") can be found in Appendix A in this volume. The full procedures for conducting an effective FBA are not complex, but they do require a degree of study and preparation and are beyond the scope of this text. Interested individuals are referred to O'Neill et al. (1997) and Watson and Steege (2003).

Case Example

The following is a hypothetical example of a FBA and subsequent positive supports and is a compilation of actual experiences, rather than those of any one school or student.

Michele was a 15-year-old, out-of-state transfer freshman at a traditional 4-year high school. By the middle of her first semester, she had received numerous detentions for threatening other students and three office referrals for aggressive behavior, including two serious brawls with other girls. The building's supportive services team convened to consider how a prevention plan of behavioral supports could be established to reduce Michele's aggressive behavior. The school psychologist was assigned to conduct a functional behavioral assessment. He first reviewed her cumulative file and all discipline records so as to identify any possible patterns, common elements, or co-occurring problems, such as academic underachievement. Additionally, the school psychologist was interested in cataloging any previous interventions and their outcomes. He supplied all of Michele's teachers with a short check sheet that allowed them to hypothesize the function that her aggression had for her and a scatter plot form to better identify times and locales of the problem behavior (see *www.pbis.org* for available forms). With these data in hand, he made an appointment to conduct functional behavioral interviews with two of Michele's teachers. The data from these assessments indicated that the afternoon classes were clearly the most high-risk environments and the classroom entry transitions the highest risk time periods within those classes. It was hypothesized that Michele brought unresolved conflicts encountered during passing time in the hallway into the classroom. A further hypothesis was that she lacked the skill necessary to moderate her anger sufficiently so as to either resolve the conflict through nonaggressive means or simply decide to ignore it entirely. The function of her aggressive behavior was rendered to this summary statement: "When Michele believes that another party has behaved toward her in a threatening or otherwise personally undesirable fashion, she responds aggressively in order to quell her anger arousal at that other party." In other words, the "pay-off" or function of her behavior is reduced anger arousal.

With those hypotheses in mind, the supportive services team worked with the classroom teachers and Michele to provide her with high levels of supervision and behavioral and emotional support at classroom entry. Michele agreed to participate in a skills training group to learn strategies for anger control and prosocial conflict resolution. In addition, the assessment uncovered failing or near-failing grades in all of her academic classes, and an emergency academic support program run through her guidance counselor was initiated. Data were collected in the form of subsequent disciplinary referrals, monitored academic progress, and student and teacher acceptability assessments to help evaluate and make modifications to the supports.

Indicated Procedures: The Needs of the Most Challenging Students

Comparatively uncomplicated and only mildly invasive supports of the kind provided to Michele in the previous example can be designed to meet the needs of most students at risk for aggressive behavior in the school setting. As noted, however, there is a third, much smaller subset of students who display chronic and severe emotional and behavioral problems in the school and who require a much more comprehensive support structure. In the three-tiered model students in this category receive *indicated prevention* programs and procedures. In most secondary school cases, these students receive curricular and behavioral programming through special education in programs for students with emotional behavioral disabilities (EBD). However, programming through EBD, in and of itself, is hardly a guarantee of adequate behavioral supports. Compared with students in general and in other special education programs, youths with EBD "have disproportionately higher rates of dropout and academic failure, and they are more likely to be arrested, poor, unemployed, involved with illicit drugs, and teen parents" (Eber et al., 2002; p. 137).

When a student with EBD is also exhibiting chronic patterns of interpersonal aggression in the secondary school setting, providing effective behavioral supports can be a daunting and, indeed, at times precarious undertaking. It appears to be no accident that the bulk of the research with aggressive students is with younger and physically smaller children. In similar fashion to students in general education receiving selected-level supports, effective behavioral supports for students with extraordinary behavioral challenges starts with a comprehensive assessment of the environmental and within-student elements that occasion the aggression. These data should drive the design and implementation of the Individualized Education Plan (IEP), a document that should be better known for its fluidity in changing circumstances than its often more typical rigidity. Mandated behavioral goals and benchmarks should be linked to research-supported interventions derived from well-constructed FBAs. When a student with EBD engages in an aggressive act in the school setting, the circumstances of the incident should serve to inform the IEP team and provide them with useful data to make modifications.

Students receiving indicated-level prevention often require the support of every resource that the school can garner. At this tier, the goals for providing knowledge and skills to prevent the onset of seriously disabling emotional problems and behavioral patterns are much more reserved than at the other two levels, and the major focus is instead on the provision of support to retard the worsening of the problem. Recent investigations by Eber and her colleagues (see Eber et al., 2002, for a review and useful discussion) have examined the use of "wraparound" services for students with EBD:

Wraparound incorporates a family-centered and strength-based philosophy of care to guide service planning for students with EBD and their families. It involves all service and strategies necessary to meet the individual needs of students and their families. The child, family members, and their team of natural support and professional providers define the needs and collectively shape and create the supports, services, and interventions linked to agreed upon outcomes. (p. 139)

Indicated prevention measures such as these figuratively "wrap" supports around the student, in and out of school, with a highly structured and individualized program (Larson et al., 2002). A team consisting of school, family, and community support individuals (e.g., family mental health professional, probation officer, social welfare worker) meet to identify student and family strengths, prioritize needs, and develop a plan for action. Support is constructed for the school, home, and community settings. Such wraparound plans may include: (1) modification of schedules, routines, and supervision; (2) skills training; (3) enhancements of existing strengths; (4) improvement of access to resources; (5) supports for caregivers; and (6) function-based behavioral supports (Eber et al., 2002). In this manner a student with what may be serious, life-course-persistent emotional and behavioral needs is provided with every available opportunity to function effectively in the traditional school environment.

Case Example

The following is a hypothetical example of a wraparound program and a compilation of actual experiences, rather than those of any one school or student.

Roger was a 12-year-old, seventh-grade student in the EBD program at a traditional grades 6–8 middle school located in a major urban area. Roger had been enrolled in special education programming since the second grade. His cumulative record was thick with IEP records and reports from numerous mental health agencies where he had at various times been diagnosed with attention-deficit/hyperactivity disorder, oppositional defiant disorder, bipolar disorder, and, most recently, conduct disorder. He has three juvenile arrests stemming from community misbehavior and one following a severe beating he inflicted upon a fellow student in school during the sixth grade. A subsequent manifestation hearing determined that his aggressive behavior was a symptom of his disability, and the public school was determined to be the least restrictive environment. He had been on court-ordered probation for 2 years. His experience in the sixth grade was characterized by unsuccessful attempts at inclusion programming that resulted in almost daily office referrals for disruptive, noncompliant, or threatening behavior.

Prior to the start of his seventh-grade year, the principal assembled a school team consisting of Roger's mother, the EBD teacher, the school psychologist, the school social worker, and the guidance counselor. These individuals further identified Roger's probation officer, the family's social caseworker, Roger's

favorite uncle, and the youth leader from the family's church as important support persons. The entire team met, and the school psychologist was designated
as the team facilitator. Goals were developed, and a comprehensive functional
behavioral assessment plan was designed. In subsequent meetings the group
developed a "wraparound" plan that opened communications and collapsed
support services in the school, home, and community into a single, unified plan
of action. In the community the uncle and the church youth leader collaborated
in efforts to provide Roger with access to more socially skilled peers in structured after-school and weekend activities. The caseworker was able to enroll
Roger's mother in a parent management training class so that she could learn to
address his behavioral needs in a more effective manner, and the school social
worker was designated the school liaison to that training and responsible for
weekly school reports to the probation officer. The school psychologist and the
EBD teacher collaborated on the development of a system of schoolwide positive
behavioral supports linked to the FBA, and the guidance counselor enrolled
Roger to her anger management training group.

SUMMARY

An argument can be raised that there is no single formula or prescription for creating
a low-aggression learning environment that is the right fit for every secondary school.
Clearly, the needs from community to community differ. The middle school my son
attended in a small college town was on almost every measure very different from the
highly urbanized middle schools I worked in as a school psychologist. Yet students
with problematic levels of aggressive behavior who disrupt the safety of the learning
environment are present in all communities, rural to urban. It is true that the perni-
cious effects of poverty and its associated risk factors weigh much more heavily on
some communities than others, catastrophically so in some cases, and this influences
the percentage of students with needs in this area to vary markedly from school to
school. However, around the country the students in every building in every school
district can be assigned a place *somewhere* on the three-tiered prevention pyramid
discussed in this chapter. It is the percentage of the whole occupied by each tier that
will represent the between-community, between-school differences, and it is those
differences that will help define the prevention mission faced by the school leadership.

The needs of schoolchildren have changed faster than the abilities of school professionals to adequately address them. It was not so long ago that schools did not
even have to accept the challenge of educating secondary-level students with diverse
learning and behavioral needs. Students either fit the existing structure or, directly or
indirectly, they were pushed out of the system. The end result was that not many
educators needed to care much about adolescent students with problem behavior

because they were either in prison, on the streets, or working in jobs—they certainly weren't raising daily havoc in the school building. That is no longer the case.

As a consequence, university research into meeting the learning and behavioral needs of an increasingly diverse student body has had to play catch-up, and there is still very much to learn. Which programs are best for which students and what combination of programs is best for which schools are questions that have yet to be answered by the empirical research literature. As this research progresses, what is currently available for concerned school personnel are emerging "best practices" recommendations. The three-tiered pyramid model discussed in this chapter provides a structure for school personnel to implement a variety of empirically supported prevention measures and to evaluate their effectiveness in the context of their individual situations.

CHAPTER 3

◆ ◆ ◆

Rationale and Best Practices for Anger and Aggression Management Skills Training

◆

A central feature of any prevention-oriented discipline program is that the adults view discipline as a process for furthering education—as a way for students to gain increased competency to manage the myriad problems they encounter both in and out of school. From this perspective, discipline should be viewed as an "instrument for student success" that is linked rationally to the mission of the school (Colvin, Kameenui, & Sugai, 1993, p. 369). The largest, most behaviorally skilled segment of the student population is provided vehicles by which to acquire new and increasingly sophisticated coping skills through universal prevention procedures such as codes of conduct and collaboratively developed classroom rules and routines. These socially competent students typically arrive at middle and high schools already possessing most of the requisite skills to allow these primary prevention programs to be useful to them. As examples:

- They have multiple, nonaggressive coping repertoires for managing frustration and perceived personal threats.
- They are experienced and adept at acquiring adult approval and willing to be deferential to adult authority.
- They are able to regulate their anger along a continuum of intensity appropriate for the situation at hand.
- They are able to inhibit impulsive behavior in conformance to a stated rule or the general mores of socially acceptable behavior.

An effective discipline program is designed to help *all* students find success. Following the spirit of the law, as well as the legal mandate of providing an appropriate public education for everyone, the needs of that subset of students who lack some or all of these skills must be addressed systematically through the use of evidence-supported procedures. Consequently, prevention-oriented anger and aggression management skills training designated for the selected subset of students with chronic patterns of disruptive, aggressive behavior must be viewed as an essential, not optional, component of every secondary school's student discipline plan (see Figure 3.1).

It is ethically and professionally indefensible for school personnel to knowingly withhold critical knowledge and skills from any group of students, including those whose behavior they may find particularly disagreeable. Individuals with chronic patterns of disruptive, aggressive behavior are students with learning needs in every bit the same way as are students with only academic deficits. Indeed, when one compares the risk status of poorly managed aggression to that of academic underachievement, a substantive argument for an even greater need for intervention can be made in favor of the former. A colleague once observed, "Who would you rather be mar-

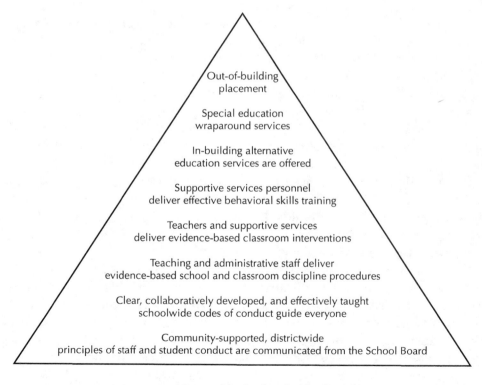

FIGURE 3.1. Pyramid of schoolwide discipline.

ried to, someone who couldn't read or someone who couldn't stop from punching you in the face?"

That said, it should also be noted that providing behaviorally at-risk youth with research-based skills training targeted to their areas of greatest deficit will not guarantee socially desirable outcomes. The data show impressively that a significant portion of adolescent aggression is the latest manifestation of a well-established trajectory begun in early childhood (Loeber, 1988, 1990; Patterson, DeBaryshe, & Ramsey, 1989), and there has been relatively limited empirical support for even the most commonly used programs (Smith, Larson, DeBaryshe, & Salzman, 2000; Tolan & Guerra, 1994). However, even as research continues, schools have an obligation to the communities, families, and students that they serve to put forward the "best practices" known and available. This chapter attempts to address those best practices and the barriers that may preclude their implementation.

WHY JUST THE THREAT OF AVERSIVE CONSEQUENCES WILL NOT WORK

Administrators are rightly concerned about keeping their buildings safe for all staff members and students. All parents want their children to be free from any form of physical and verbal assault while they are in school and expect the building administrator to ensure that they are. The powers are granted to most administrators to unilaterally decide which incidences of student misconduct are grievous enough to warrant temporary removal from the school; therefore, it is understandable that the most common disciplinary response to aggressive behavior has been found to be out-of-school suspension (e.g., Costenbader & Markson, 1994). If the potential assailants are not physically in the building, then their ability to assault others is removed, at least for the short term. In behavioral terms, an action such as suspension out of school is negatively reinforced (see Kazdin, 2001) when it removes or terminates the aversive condition of the presence of disruptive or aggressive students. In this manner, suspension works . . . at least for the administrator. Indeed, for some it apparently works exceedingly well: In the year 2000 administrators in the Milwaukee Public Schools suspended out of school *fully 20% of their student population*, most for nonaggressive behaviors (Milwaukee Catalyst, 2001).

The research that demonstrates the negative effects of out-of-school suspension is impressive (see Skiba, 2000, for a review). However, even educators who are the most enthusiastically against out-of-school suspension will acknowledge that some circumstances may warrant it, especially those situations that require immediate protection of the individuals involved with no other way to accomplish it. Removing a student to a safe and supervised home situation for a brief "cooling-off" period can be constructive in some cases. The operative word, of course, is "supervised," and given the dual-wage-earner status of most homes, supervision is rarely available. Students who are out of school unsupervised are at high risk to engage in community juvenile crime (National Criminal Justice Reference Service, n.d.).

Many of us can recall as children and adolescents being the recipients of some manner of threat-based coercion from our parents used as a mechanism to obtain compliance. This age-old parenting technique most often took the form of: (1) a conditional proposition ("If you aren't in by midnight . . . ") followed by (2) an aversive consequence (" . . . then you are grounded the rest of the weekend"). This method of offspring control is based on the well-established principle that individuals will alter their behavior in order to avoid an aversive consequence (Kazdin, 2001). The comparative effectiveness of this disciplinary technique hinges on four suppositions:

1. *There is an evident and genuine power and authority hierarchy.* If family membership is comprised of a recognized hierarchy, beginning with the parents and moving downward to the children, then the adolescent is able to recognize the moral authority of the parents to create such conditions.

2. *The adolescent finds the proposed consequence aversive.* For most adolescents, effective removal of previously enjoyed and anticipated freedoms through grounding is indeed aversive; hence its widespread use as a parent-issued consequence.

3. *The adolescent believes that the consequence will be carried out unfailingly.* If the offending adolescent believes that his parents are "all hat and no cattle" (as my Texas friends say) and easily talked out of it, then the anticipated aversive nature of the consequence disappears, along with its power to influence behavior.

4. *The adolescent has the requisite cognitive, emotional, and behavioral characteristics to understand and adhere to the proposition.* As the curfew time approaches, if the adolescent lacks the intellectual ability for consequential thinking, or the ability to regulate his or her anger at having to interrupt a reinforcing condition, or the behavioral or attentional skills to manage time effectively, then the power of the remote consequence to influence compliance to authority is reduced or absent.

In a fashion similar to families, schools have the obligation to make reasonable compliance demands on the students and to organize discipline structures to increase the likelihood of their observance. The *effective* use of remote aversive consequences by school personnel (e.g., exclusion procedures of expulsion, suspension, detention) to increase student compliance to codified behavioral expectations hinges on the same four presuppositions noted earlier for adolescents in a family. Although it is entirely possible that some students inhibit aggressive behavior out of fear of the consequence of exclusion, there is no empirical data to support this proposition (Skiba, 2000). Let us see how the four essential presuppositions apply to a school policy that asserts,"If you engage in aggressive behavior, then you will be excluded (suspended, expelled) from school."

1. *There is an evident and genuine power and authority hierarchy.* Sprick (1998) hypothesized that chronically disruptive students may tend to see themselves and all adults in the school as occupying the same spot on the authority hierarchy. He proposed that for many such youths, an interaction with any adult in the building— secretary, teacher, counselor, administrator—holds virtually equal meaning and that a referral from teacher to administrator is more a *lateral* than an *ascending* move up any presumed hierarchical discipline structure. Indeed, Sprick's notion was that these students internally place themselves on equal social status with the adults, thus denying the legitimacy of a teacher or administrator to direct their behavior in any way. In other words, many chronically disruptive students may not even recognize the school's authority to implement a disciplinary procedure as a result of a firmly held "You can't tell me what to do" belief structure. Although there is no current research that supports this hypothesis, it has undeniable clinical appeal and offers a reasonable explanation for the failure of many students to be at all deterred by the prospect of an administrative referral.

2. *The adolescent finds the proposed consequence aversive.* Exclusionary discipline procedures such as out-of-school suspension are predicated on the supposition that the student actually *wants* to be in school and will be distressed to be excluded, even for a short period. It is altogether possible that a subset of aggressive, disruptive adolescents would be upset at the prospect of 3 days out of school, particularly when the event triggers a home consequence of greater aversion. However, unlike their more academically involved peers, the "fear" of missing classes and sleeping in late for 3 days does not hold the same sway for most students with chronic disruptive aggression. For a great percentage of these individuals, their school experience is defined by Bob Dylan's line, "When you ain't got nothin', you got nothin' to lose."

3. *The adolescent believes that the consequence will be carried out unfailingly.* When the consequence is not aversive but, indeed, may be desirable, holding this belief may be more of an incentive than a deterrent. "Zero tolerance" policies that eliminate the ability of the administrator to enact an individualized, educational, or even more aversive consequence and instead force a suspension may be working counter to their intent (e.g., Skiba & Peterson, 1999).

4. *The adolescent has the requisite cognitive, emotional, and behavioral characteristics to understand and adhere to the proposition.* When a student is presented with the opportunity and motivation to enact a behavior that has been previously reinforced, such as punching a peer who, one believes, deserves it, the ability to inhibit this behavior out of fear of a consequence coming later requires that this student possess a rather sophisticated degree of cognitive-emotive control. Not only must the young person find the remote consequences aversive in the first place (an issue previously addressed), but he or she must simultaneously be able to regulate escalating anger and control impulse behavior while selecting and enacting an alternative, nonaggressive response. Difficulties with affect regulation, impulse control,

and response selection are characteristics frequently seen in individuals with aggressive behavior (Dodge, 1991; Dodge et al., 1990; Lochman, Meyer, et al., 1991; Novaco, 1985). When a discipline policy makes continuance in school contingent on a set of skills that some students do not possess, the results are predictable. As an example, I can put you in front of a disassembled color television set and threaten you with all manner of terrible, escalating consequences if you don't immediately put it back together correctly. My threats are meaningless if you do not have the skills necessary to do so, and I shouldn't be surprised if you got up and walked away. In the same fashion, an administrator or a Board of Education can increase the severity of the consequence for aggression all they want, but if the student does not know how to behave—*if that student lacks the prerequisite skills to adhere to the policy*—then no level of severity will be sufficient.

WHY ALTERNATIVE AVERSIVE CONSEQUENCES ARE NOT ENOUGH

A growing number of middle and high schools, perhaps heeding the research literature, have begun experimenting with aversive disciplinary consequences that do not involve out-of-school suspensions. Typically these consequences involve some form of in-school suspension, Saturday school, or after-school detentions (Morgan-D'Atrio, Northrup, LaFleur, & Spera, 1996). These efforts constitute a double-edged sword. In the case of in-school suspension, although students are excluded from the classroom, they remain under competent adult supervision, which eliminates the possibility of community misbehavior during school hours. The positives associated with this alternative should not be underestimated. An administrator colleague remarked to me that sending chronically misbehaving students into the community for 3 to 5 days "only gives them practice in what to do and who to hang out with when they drop out."

Second, when a school replaces out-of-school suspension with in-school suspension, a considerably diminished rejection message is relayed. The misbehaving student is informed that although the behavior is unacceptable and will have a negative consequence, the education personnel believe that the student rightly belongs and is welcome in the school building. This simple message may contribute to helping high-risk youths maintain a sense, even if tenuous, of belonging to the school, and this cognitive-emotional bond has been shown to be a critical factor in both violence and dropout prevention (Hawkins et al., 1992).

The negative edge of this double-edged sword lies in the belief that the somewhat progressive and enlightened step of replacing out-of-school suspension with in-school suspension is a sufficient adjustment to meet the needs of all students. It is not. Aversive consequences, educationally benign or not, do not teach new and complex coping skills to unskilled youths. Offending students with chronic patterns of aggressive behavior who are doing work sheets in the in-school suspension room may be inconvenienced and are probably longing to be elsewhere, but they are assuredly not learning the skills needed to avoid coming back another day.

Nor does the addition of some form of written or verbal reflection on the incident serve a useful purpose for such needy students. Many in-school suspension programs, seeking to move beyond simple aversive boredom as their consequence, require that the students engage in a "behavioral debriefing" procedure with the adult in charge. This well-intentioned exercise may provide the student with insight into his or her responsibility for the problem, and he or she may even go on to discuss alternative behaviors that might have been enacted to avoid the problem. Presumably, there is hope that the student will take these insights away from the discussion and use them to avoid future difficulties. For chronically aggressive and behaviorally unskilled students, however, some may assert that this exercise is akin to "giving chicken soup to a corpse: It can't hurt." But it *can* hurt if the school personnel believe that merely providing guided insight for these students is an "intervention" and if they subsequently move to more exclusionary discipline measures when the students "fail to respond." The implementation of well-meaning but inadequate, empirically unsupported disciplinary interventions is among the greatest barriers to success faced by high-risk students.

BEST PRACTICES

As noted, the implementation of purely reactive disciplinary procedures to meet the behavioral needs of chronically aggressive middle and high school students is unlikely to be sufficient. In-school aversive consequences must be paired with an additional preventative educational component that effectively teaches the cognitive and behavioral skills necessary for success in the school environment. The following are essential components of that education.

Anger Management

Not all adolescent assaults in the school are fueled by anger, but for those students with chronic patterns of aggression that have been unresponsive to traditional reactive disciplinary measures, aggression often follows poorly regulated anger arousal (Feindler & Ecton, 1986). Consequently, helping students to understand and control anger is a particularly important skills training component.

The following useful definition of anger was offered by Kassinove and Sukhodolsky (1995): "a negative, phenomenological (or internal) feeling state associated with specific cognitive and perceptual distortions and deficiencies (e.g., mis-appraisals, errors and attributions of blame, injustice, preventability and/or intentionality), subjective labeling, physiological changes, and action tendencies to engage in socially constructed and reinforced behavioral scripts" (p. 7). This definition highlights the three most salient elements of the anger experience—physiological, cognitive, and behavioral—the understanding of which is essential to the task of anger control and must be addressed in any skills-training effort.

The hypothesized causal relationship that anger may or may not have to aggression has been the subject of considerable study and opinion. Some researchers (most notably Berkowitz, 1993) hold that angry feelings do not directly cause aggression but rather that they accompany an already existing inclination to aggression. It is clear that some adolescents who are aggressive do not display any obvious signs of anger. Bully behavior, as an example, is most frequently seen as physical or verbal aggression directed at a less powerful victim, but it is rarely motivated by poorly controlled anger (Olweus, 1991; but see also Bosworth, Espelage, & Simon, 1999, for research on a possible anger correlate). This sort of aggressive behavior, designed to obtain some manner of goal (e.g., victim humiliation) but rarely motivated by anger, has been referred to as *instrumental aggression* (e.g., Spielberger, Reheiser, & Sydeman, 1995) or *proactive aggression* (Dodge, 1991). Many bullies and other student aggressors of this type typically do not have serious anger control problems and may instead be more responsive to interventions that involve increased supervision and aversive consequences. Acts of aggression that are heavily influenced by anger control problems have been referred to as *hostile aggression* (e.g., Spielberger, Reheiser, & Sydeman, 1995) or *reactive aggression* (Dodge, 1991). This is the kind of student aggression typically precipitated by the intense physiological arousal and cognitive distortions described in Kassinove and Sukhodolsky's (1995) definition of anger noted earlier, and these are the students who may benefit most from anger control training.

This dichotomous, reactive–proactive conceptualization of aggressive types is useful for educators as they consider the potential environmental and individual variables associated with any act of student aggression. However, it is important to recognize that these are very rarely pure types, except in extreme cases. "All behaviors have aspects of reaction and proaction, in that one can make guesses regarding the precipitants as well as the functions of all behaviors" (Dodge, 1991, p. 206). Caution is recommended against the inclination to oversimplify this helpful, but still theoretical, construct by wrongly labeling students as just one or the other. The student targeted for anger control training, however, will demonstrate predominantly reactive aggressive characteristics.

Meichenbaum (2001) described reactive aggression in the following manner:

Impulsive aggression, often called *reactive aggression*, is <u>unplanned</u> aggressive acts which are <u>spontaneous</u> in action: either <u>unprovoked</u> or <u>out of proportion</u> to the provocation and occurs among persons who are characterized as *"having a short fuse."* Such *reactive aggression* involves retaliatory intent, often driven by frustration, biological impulses and relatively independent of premeditated cognitive processes. (p. 20; emphasis in original)

Middle and high school students who exhibit this kind of "short fuse" aggressive response to what appears to be only minor provocation by peers or adults are the primary targets for anger control training. Helping students learn to curb this short fuse requires that the training address the three elements of impulsive anger—poorly regulated physiological responses, distorted cognitions, and aggressive behavior. With that understanding, the following procedures are the essential elements of a school-based anger and aggression control program, presented in the recommended order of training. It is important to note that the procedures introduced here and expanded on later in this book are cognitive-behavioral skills training, not "psychotherapy" in its traditional conceptualization. They focus on elements in the current environment and existing social-cognitive skill deficits that occasion anger and aggression rather than hypothesizing about and addressing remote causes.

Anger and Aggression Education

The initial step in an anger and aggression control program is to provide the students with intellectual insight into the nature and function of both anger and aggression. This is done so that everyone in the group has as close to a common understanding as possible when the terms are utilized in the training weeks to come. The group examines and proposes their own definitions of "healthy anger" that helps avoid unwanted problems with significant others (e.g., teachers, administrators, police, parents) and may lead to desirable, productive change. This is compared with "unhealthy anger" that is more intense than warranted by the situation and that may lead to unwanted problems with significant others. An essential aspect of understanding their experience of anger is acquiring the insight that the intensity of the feeling runs a continuum from mild irritation to their more familiar highly intense experience. How an individual labels a feeling is critical to his or her understanding and control of it. If the students conceptualize anger *only* as their typical rage response, then "being angry" can only mean being enraged. This aspect of the affective education procedures seeks to normalize human anger, and the students are introduced to a functional vocabulary (e.g., "irritated," "peeved," "put out") to label less intense feelings.

Students are subsequently led toward a functional definition of aggression, including physical, verbal, and relational types. Insights into the subject of aggression are shared, such as how posture and language can be construed as aggressive acts by others and when and where physical aggression may be in the students' best interests. Finally, the students are led to insights regarding the relationship between unhealthy anger and aggression.

Cue Recognition and Self-Calming

"How do you know that you are becoming angry?" Although it may be the first time anyone ever posed the question, individuals without anger problems will often readily reply with answers such as: "I can feel my face become flushed," or "I can feel my heart start to accelerate." Such individuals who are able to regulate the intensity of their anger under multiple conditions are generally able to answer that question with little difficulty. This is so because their ability to exercise the necessary control starts with a phenomenological recognition of the feeling: They know what their own anger feels like, and that feeling serves as a cue to exert their control mechanisms. This phenomenological self-awareness is often a much greater problem for students with chronic, anger-related aggression.

One reason that this ability may be a problem for such students is simply that they have seldom felt the need to control their anger. Their answer to the question "How do you know that you are becoming angry?" very often brings forth a behavior rather than an internal feeling: *"Because I start hitting the guy."* These adolescents know that they are angry when they are up in a teacher's face or pummeling a fellow student with their fists. The time between the state of nonanger and the state of rage is often so slight as to make the whole notion of "escalating" anger almost meaningless to them. Yet in order to learn control of their anger, their first step is to learn recognition of those initial physiological cues.

Tied closely to cue recognition is the first training in anger control, what is referred to as "self-calming" procedures. The students are trained in simple relaxation methods (e.g., controlled breathing) or refocusing procedures (e.g., backward counting) to quickly, but only temporarily, control the escalating intensity as preparation for additional skill enactments to follow.

Attribution Retraining

One of the most important cognitive skills of nonaggressive individuals is their ability to effectively read a variety of social cues and consider multiple attributions for the behavior of others. Attributions are the individual's explanation to himself or herself regarding the intent of another's actions. If you bump into me and I attribute your action to benign carelessness, then I am unlikely to become upset. In essence, I am telling myself to remain calm and that there is no reason to become angry. On the other hand, if I attribute it to a hostile act on your part, a wholly different feeling may ensue. Research with aggressive children and adolescents (e.g., Crick & Dodge, 1994; Dodge et al., 1990) has demonstrated that biased attributions play a role in reactive aggression.

The term "hostile attributional bias" (Dodge & Newman, 1981; Nasby, Hayden, & DePaulo, 1979) has been used to describe a cognitive process in which aggressive individuals regularly interpret the behavior of others as hostile, even in situations that are benign or ambiguous. Kendall et al. (1991) referred to this as the "tendency to 'assume the worst' regarding the intention of peers in ambiguous (neither hostile nor benign) situations" (p. 345). Exploration of this tendency (e.g., Dodge & Tomlin, 1987; Hudley, 1994) has led to the hypothesis that such a bias is in part a function of the individual's tendency "to respond based on past experience rather than all available social cues" (Hudley, 1994, p. 45). In other words, aggressive students may lack the skill to access critical information when engaged in decision-making strategies. This is a critical feature of anger control training because the probability and intensity of anger increases if the action is judged intentional (Deffenbacher, 1999).

Consider Michael, a very hot-headed and aggressive eighth-grade student, who is eating with a group of fellow students in the school lunchroom. The student sitting next to him tips his milk carton over, and some of its contents pour onto Michael's lap, not an uncommon occurrence in middle school lunchrooms. This is a benign or at least ambiguous encounter up to this point. Metaphorically speaking, the ball is now in Michael's court to infer intent for the spillage. Youths with high levels of reactive aggression have a greater than typical expectation that others will be hostile toward them. Consequently, they are hypervigilant for confirming evidence. For Michael the milk on his trousers is just such evidence.

A less aggressive student might immediately start a search for environmental cues that would help him determine whether the milk on his pants was the result of an accident or a hostile act. For most nonaggressive youths, the default inference in such circumstances is "accident," and they are alert for those expected social cues. A subsequent nonaggressive behavioral response characteristically follows. When an attribution of hostile intent is missing, then the likelihood of aggression diminishes. In secondary-level schools, this typically benign student attribution for the multitude of minute-to-minute interpersonal transgressions may be a major reason that the school can function at all!

But for students such as Michael, the default attribution is not accident but hostility, a purposeful, aggressive act. This expectation is so strong that Michael will ignore current, relevant social cues to the contrary (e.g., quick apologies, offers of a napkin) and rely much more heavily on his memory of previous similar encounters either with this student or in this context. He infers intent, and his behavioral response is aggressive. He swears at his perceived attacker and shoves him. The other student, who is now the recipient of a clearly aggressive act, moves into an equally clear counteraggressive posture and rises to meet Michael's aggression. This counteraggressive behavior has the effect of confirming for Michael that his original attribution of hostility was accurate, and, thus, it is reinforced. Another lunchroom fracas is on.

Attribution re-training to assist students at risk for aggressive behavior has been demonstrated to have positive outcomes with elementary-age boys (Hudley, 1992; Hudley et al., 1998; see Chapter 1, this volume). No research to date has been undertaken to examine similar effects on middle or high school students, and this is a serious gap in the literature. The basic research data (e.g., Dodge et al., 1990) offer compelling evidence that attributions play a significant role in the frequency and intensity of anger-induced reactive aggression in both children and adolescents. Consequently, the inclusion of a component to address this process in an anger control training program for adolescents is clinically warranted, even ahead of the applied research. Insight is provided into the fact that anger does not "just happen" but is heavily related to how a student individually chooses to appraise a situation and the relative accuracy of that appraisal. The training elements utilize role play and "think aloud" procedures in conjunction with hypothetical and actual scenarios to help the students learn to consider alternative attributions.

Self-Instructional Training

Training middle and high school adolescents with anger and aggression control problems to "talk to themselves" is an essential component of an effective program. The concept of teaching self-instruction as an intervention to guide behavior originated with Meichenbaum and Goodman (1971) in their classic work with impulsive children. Since that time, it has established a solid place in the clinical treatment of children, adolescents, and adults with anger control problems (e.g., Feindler & Ecton, 1986; Feindler, Ecton, Kingsley, & Dubey, 1986; Feindler, Marriott, & Iwata, 1984; Larson, 1992; Lochman, White, & Wayland, 1991; Meichenbaum, 2001). Self-instructional training is a technique that provides the youth with a cognitive alternative to his or her more characteristic biased, distorted, or deficient script. As noted by Rokke and Rehm (2001), "An explicit assumption is that an individual's self-instructions mediate behavior and behavior change. In many cases maladaptive self-statements may contribute to a person's problems. The learning and application of more adaptive self-instructions are the goals of self-instructional training" (p. 178). Meichenbaum (2001, p. 281) addressed the differential uses of self-instruction during the phases of an anger encounter:

- Preparing for the stressful encounters and getting worked up (anticipating provocative event).
- Having to deal with perceived provocation and confrontations.
- Dealing with anger at its most intense point.
- Reflecting back on how they handled the situation.

During these meetings students are further trained in the concept introduced in attribution retraining regarding how their own internal language can influence their anger to escalate or moderate in intensity. Self-instructional training provides the students with suggested self-statements that have been used by other adolescents (e.g., "Cool down"; "Chill out"; "I can handle this") and also encourages the students to tap their own vocabularies to develop more individualized coping statements. Through role play and self-monitoring procedures, training focuses on helping the students to effectively identify the circumstances and timing for the use of self-instruction as an anger control procedure.

Problem-Solving Skills Training

For you, the predominantly high-achieving professionals and graduate students who are the readers of this book, the likelihood is great that you possess impressive problem-solving abilities. On a regular basis, you encounter situations of ambiguity, possible threat, or provocation and somehow manage to find an adaptive response. Imagine a situation in which you are driving along a four-lane highway and another driver cuts in front of you, causing you to have to brake quickly. Almost instantaneously, you address the problem by backing off from the intruding vehicle and continuing your drive (perhaps muttering a few choice words). This is the adaptive response of individuals without problematic anger and aggression, and it is the result of a well-learned problem-solving strategy. In this case (1) you recognized the problem, (2) considered your options, (3) weighed their relative merits, (4) selected the best response, and (5) enacted it, all in the blink of an eye. This highly adaptive, cognitive-behavioral skill that you employ with regularity across multiple contexts and among multiple individuals may be one of the primary reasons you are not reading these words from a prison cell.

The impulsive anger and aggression responses that characterize reactive-aggressive youths necessarily preclude or seriously undermine the application of systematic problem-solving strategies. Highly aggressive children and adolescents have been shown to demonstrate biased appraisal of hostile intent (Crick & Dodge, 1994; Dodge et al., 1990), deficient solution-generating skills (Lochman & Dodge, 1994), and more physically aggressive responses (Pepler, Craig, & Michaels, 1998; Slaby & Guerra, 1988). Problem-solving training is the logical next step in the effort to assist identified students to better manage their problematic anger and aggression.

The goal of problem-solving training is to help the identified students perceive the myriad provocations they encounter in the school day as *problems to be solved* (Meichenbaum, 2001) rather than *personal assaults* to be settled with aggression. This is approached by teaching the students to conceptualize the problem as a sequential series of skills in stepwise form, including "(1) problem definition and formulation, (2) generation of alternative solutions, (3) decision-making, and (4) solution implementation and verification" (D'Zurilla & Nezu, 1999, p. 215).

As an example, consider a hypothetical circumstance in which a student is unfairly accused of cheating by his teacher, who snatches his test off his desk.

1. *What is the problem?* Students are taught to step back (sometimes even literally) and define the problem in terms of their own participation and their own goals.

"The problem is the teacher thinks I was cheating, but I wasn't. I want to be able to finish my test and not get sent out."

2. *What are my possible responses?* In this step the students are asked to generate as many feasible responses as they can that will address the problem and help them to obtain their desired goal.

"I could grab the paper back and tell her she was wrong."
"I could ask other students if they saw me cheating."
"I could ask her if I could talk to her in private."

3. *What will happen if . . . ?* Students are asked to reflect on the most likely consequences of each of the responses they generated. Skills associated with consequential thinking are also trained at this juncture.

"If I grab it, she will probably get even more upset and throw me out for that!"
"If I ask for witnesses, she won't like to be shown-up by the other kids and might get angrier."
"If I see her in private, she might be willing to listen. At least I won't make things worse."

4. *Which one will I choose?* At this step students need to select a response that is in their best interest based on their assessment of the most likely consequences and one that they have the necessary skills to enact.

"I will ask her if we can speak in private at her desk."

5. *How did it work out?* This step involves training the students to use self-reinforcement if the selected response was successful and self-coaching if it was not. Students need to learn how to recognize and be proud of their successful efforts and also acquire the skills needed to cope with and learn from failures.

Behavioral Skills Training

It has been said that *knowing about* the correct behavior is not the same thing as understanding how to actually *engage in* the correct behavior. Learning a novel behavior requires not only intellectual insight but also correct practice. One can observe an accomplished pianist play a Scott Joplin rag and understand that he or she is reading the notes on the sheet music and reassigning the written notes to finger movements on the keyboard. This is simple intellectual insight or knowing about the behavior. But for a novice pianist, it would take many hours of correct practice to actually demonstrate the behavior of playing a Joplin rag. In the same way, students with reactive–aggressive behavior patterns absolutely must move beyond simply knowing about new, prosocial behaviors to actively engaging in the correct practice of them. In my clinical experience, I have observed that the failure of otherwise accomplished therapists to unrelentingly engage this "practice principle" with reactively aggressive youths is the most prominent variable in poor counseling outcomes. Knowing about the uses of self-instruction or knowing about uses of verbal assertion is necessary, but not sufficient, to obtain the desired behavioral changes.

In effective skills training, the students are not merely passive recipients of insights and suggestions; they spend much of their training period up on their feet practicing new skills or engaging in behavioral rehearsal for an anticipated provocation or stressor. Behavioral skills training permeates the entire intervention and is based on the knowledge that (1) the students first need to learn how to perform the new behavior in the group setting, (2) they need to then learn how to generalize the new behavior to the authentic setting, and (3) they need to ultimately assimilate the new behavior into their regular coping repertoires. Given the risk status of highly aggressive adolescents, this is indeed a daunting set of goals. Yet if there is a perfect setting in which to make the effort, it is the public school.

Why School-Based Training?

Schools are ideal settings in which to undertake the effort of helping adolescents with anger and aggression problems, in large part because the task aligns well with the functions of the institution, that is, teaching and learning. Skills training of this sort contains many elements similar to those of traditional course work: a licensed adult in charge, students with learning needs and behavioral expectations, a curriculum in the form of a training manual, and explicit goals and objectives. The business of middle and high schools is to provide students with the knowledge and skills to be successful in and out of the academic venue, and that is entirely consonant with the business of those who seek to provide behavioral management knowledge and skills to high-risk students. In addition, the following elements argue for school-based training:

- Critical assessment data can be easily gathered through existing school record review, direct observation methods, or functional behavioral assessment interviews with classroom teachers, requiring less reliance on client self-report.
- Progress-monitoring data in the form of teacher reports, truancy reports, discipline referrals, and other authentic data can be acquired on an hourly basis if need be.
- Schoolwide and classroom environmental factors, such as positive behavioral supports and effective aversive consequences, can be influenced and manipu-

lated during training to assist the intervention and lead to improved understanding of student needs.

- Classrooms and other social–academic settings in the school provide rich and abundant opportunities for student clients to observe prosocial models and engage in authentic-setting rehearsal strategies;
- The presence of a large cadre of other education professionals (teachers, administrators, and pupil services personnel) affords opportunities for trainer consultation, collaboration, and, when needed, personal support.

Summary

Addressing the academic, social, and emotional needs of all students who attend the public school system is a Herculean but legally and ethically mandated obligation. Meeting those needs for students with aggressive behavior problems requires that school personnel advance significantly beyond traditional offerings and implement creative, even extraordinary, measures and programs. Students who engage in anger-induced aggressive behavior that has been unresponsive to ordinary discipline and administrative reactions create a volatile condition that the school must address. Included with the obligation to protect other students and staff members is the obligation to provide these very high-risk students with the knowledge and skills they need to become productive citizens.

The knowledge and skills to effectively control aggressive anger responses cannot be learned at home while on out-of-school suspension. Nor can they be learned in an at-risk academic support program or an in-school suspension or after-school detention room. In order to address the needs of reactive-aggressive youths, school personnel must commit to the addition of a targeted skills-training program that focuses on the research-supported cognitive and behavioral deficits of these students. Intervention efforts that vary remarkably from this model, including insight-oriented counseling and classroom-based anger management curricula, are not supported in the literature as being effective. For administrators and pupil services personnel this effort will require that existing discipline, intervention, and staff training priorities be reexamined and personnel resources reallocated.

CHAPTER 4

◆ ◆ ◆

Screening, Identification, and Assessment for Anger and Aggression Management Training

◆

Every morning during the school year, students arrive at middle and high schools with the full range of academic, behavioral, emotional, and physical/medical needs, and it is the job of secondary-level educators to see that those needs are met in the most efficient and effective manner possible. This is an enormous and complex task that gets increasingly difficult as the diversity of these needs expands. Pupil services personnel are often spread thin with activities such as teen parenting classes, AIDS prevention education, gang-resistance-skills training, substance abuse prevention, grief counseling, and bully and harassment prevention all added onto their more traditional and equally important duties. Consequently, when the school system mandates that the needs of students with serious anger and aggression problems also be addressed, there is an implied demand that economy of time and effort be maximized. It is a rare adolescent who could not benefit from at least some instruction in the area of anger management. How do educators determine which students should receive specific skills training? Because two students get into a fight in the lunchroom, should they automatically be placed on the list? What if a concerned parent calls asking for help with her temper-prone daughter who has been destroying her bedroom in fits of rage? This chapter is concerned with the important issues associated with ensuring that the students who are identified and selected for anger and aggression management training are those most likely to achieve the greatest benefit from it. Decisions that are this important need to be driven by forethought and available data and not by impulse or frustration.

SCREENING AND IDENTIFICATION

At the secondary level, the extent of the need for selected prevention services such as anger and aggression management skills training groups is in direct relationship to (1) the risk status of the student population as a whole, (2) the quality of the prevention program in the lower level feeder schools, and (3) the quality of the universal prevention programs within which the training is embedded. Professionals working in middle and high schools located in neighborhoods of high poverty and social disorganization must provide services for students who typically have more risk factors for negative psychosocial outcomes than the students served by their colleagues in wealthier neighborhoods (Patterson et al., 1989; Tolan, Guerra, & Kendall, 1995; Walker et al., 2004). In addition, when elementary-level prevention programs are ineffectual or absent altogether, the potential pool of high-risk students entering secondary education is broadened to include those who may have been helped at an earlier age by strong universal and selected prevention programs. Finally, the need for anger and aggression management skills training is likely to be greater in secondary schools in which evidence-supported schoolwide and classroom-level universal prevention programs are missing or poorly enacted.

The following section contains a rationally conceived risk-status heuristic designed to assist secondary-level educators in deciding which students need anger and aggression management skills training (see Table 4.1). The pool of students who

TABLE 4.1. Categorical Organization of Students with Needs for Anger and Aggression Management Skills Training

Category I: Need Determined by the Archival Behavioral Record
- Antisocial behavior patterns/disruptive school behavior from early elementary school
- Evidence of resistance to ordinary school discipline structures
- Evidence of systematic intervention efforts
- Frequent aggressive behavior patterns continuing at previous grade level

Category II: Need Determined by Resistance to High-Quality Discipline Structures
- Aggressive behavior in school history, including most recent grade level
- Chronicity not as long and frequency not as high as Category I
- Inadequate evidence of resistance to high quality discipline structures
- Demonstrates continued aggression with high quality discipline structure in new school

Caregory III: Need Determined by Individual Assessment
- Little or no history of serious aggressive behavior
- Sudden onset of aggressive behavior unexplained by obvious circumstances
- Comprehensive evaluation determines anger/aggression management to be first treatment priority

have potential need for this additional behavioral skills training over and above their inclusion in the general disciplinary structure is grouped into three categories, from those with the greatest need to those with the least. It is, by design, simple and thus open to disagreement on that count. More sophisticated and potentially more valid and reliable measures involving broad-scale multiple-gating procedures and systematic psychometric screening can be designed. Such procedures may be best for schools that have the personnel and budget to make this substantial effort on a year-to-year basis. The course of action offered here attempts to bridge the gap between that level of sophistication and no process at all and, by doing so, to potentially improve the likelihood of services being made available for those students who need them most.

Category I: Need Determined by the Archival Behavioral Record

Screening and identification procedures designed to ascertain which students will benefit from a selected prevention program in anger and aggression management at the secondary level differ from those at the elementary level. With younger students, the systematic identification of research-supported risk markers and precursor behaviors is the sine qua non of the prevention effort (see Walker et al., 2004, for an excellent discussion of these issues). Preschool- and early-primary-level students are watched carefully for behaviors and personal characteristics that have been shown to be associated with later antisocial behavior, including aggression, and proactive prevention programs are implemented. Because these precursor variables may not necessarily be "aggressive" in nature (e.g., noncompliance, fearlessness, negative emotionality; see Dannemiller, 2003), knowledge of the risk markers and application of valid and reliable identification processes are essential. Secondary schools receive the benefits of effective screening and prevention programs at the previous levels.

If the elementary school has had an active prevention program in place, by the time students reach middle school, a wealth of data is generally available to assist the new school in the effort to provide necessary behavioral and emotional supports. These data are critical. As noted in Chapter 2, fifth-grade students who have had patterns of frequent aggressive behavior in elementary school are highly likely to continue those patterns into the middle school sixth grade in much the same way that eighth-grade students are likely to continue their aggressive behavior into the ninth. Educators at entry-level middle and high schools need to abandon their well-meaning but behaviorally naive versions of "wipe the slate clean" or "fresh start." It is one thing to be nonprejudicial but quite another to ignore good science that begs educators to consider established past antisocial behaviors as healthy predictors of future behavior (e.g., Lipsey & Derzon, 1998). Attending to behavioral histories is particularly important for those students who can be seen to have "life-course-persistent antisocial behavior" (Moffitt, 1993) or are what Patterson and colleagues referred to as "early starters" (see Patterson, Reid, & Dishion, 1992, for a discussion). This research suggests that boys who start their antisocial behavior early in life are at significantly greater risk to become chronic offenders than those who do not begin until later in adolescence. The behavioral records that arrive with incoming students are an essential data source to be carefully reviewed by the next level of educators. The simple transition to another level of schooling is not an intervention: There is no preceding "magic summer" that changes risk status.

Category I students arrive at the middle or high school with clear and compelling needs for anger and aggression management training and positive behavioral supports. Whether they are receiving services under IDEA or within general education is irrelevant to those needs. The mere act of determining that a student is a "child with a disability" in no way diminishes the obligation of the school to provide the necessary skills for success. A special education support classroom or the services of an inclusion teacher is generally insufficient to meet this obligation. Special education students who lack the skills to manage their own reactive aggression will continue this behavior as long as it is reinforced and as long as they continue to lack the knowledge and skills to invoke alternative responses. In this manner they are no different from their general education counterparts.

The effort to determine who the potential Category I students are in an incoming class of students should begin in the spring of the year preceding the transition to middle or high school. The defining risk features of a Category I student are as follows:

1. There is documentation of chronic, frequent, overt antisocial behavior, including non-compliance, oppositional behavior, and aggression in the school setting, dating to earlier in elementary school and continuing into the present school year.
2. There is documentation of the systematic implementation of evidence-supported prevention and intervention measures designed to address the student's specific behavioral needs. These measures must go well beyond ordinary exclusionary discipline and parent contacts and include selected prevention procedures such as behavioral skills training and schoolwide positive behavioral supports.

The following are essential questions for the receiving school to have answered (see Appendix A: "Current Behavior Screening Form"):

- Has the student been receiving research-supported anger and aggression skills training at the previous school? It is helpful to think of such interventions as "coping supports" rather than efforts at a "cure." *Continuation of that support is almost always warranted unless there is convincing evidence to the contrary.* A student's having difficulties in spite of the ongoing intervention is not sufficient evidence of its lack of value. The experience of the intervention may be the primary reason that the problems did not become worse.

- What other behavioral supports were effective? This is the essential question asked to avoid wasting time, effort, and expense to "reinvent the wheel." In addition to continued skills training, were there other environmental supports that increased the likelihood of adaptive conflict resolution and that can be implemented at the next level? For instance, if the availability of a "cool down" room was effective previously, it is wise to have it in place on opening day. On the other hand, if weekly report cards to parents served only to aggravate an already dysfunctional home situation, an alternative or revised home–school collaboration system should be designed.
- What do classroom teachers need to know and be able to do to work effectively with this student? Middle and high school teachers should not have to discover the presence of a highly volatile student on their own. A preclass consultation with a knowledgeable pupil services staff member is critically important to avoid "surprises." Previous teachers are gold mines of information, and efforts to tap that resource generally pay off well. Helpful information, such as about common classroom anger triggers, instructional levels and effective methods, and curricular adaptations, can all help to ease the transition.

Category I students represent that population of incoming or newly transferred middle and high school students whose needs for anger and aggression skills training are virtually unquestionable. For these students, taking a "wait and see" posture in the face of compelling data to the contrary is poor educational practice, and for mental health professionals in the schools, it is professionally unethical (Jacob & Hartshorne, 2003).

Category II: Need Determined by Resistance to High-Quality Discipline Structures

Category II is a grouping of students who may have evident risk status but for whom, as newly entering students, there are reasonable grounds to hold off the immediate implementation of anger and aggression skills training. The young person may have a problematic behavioral record from his or her previous grade level or school, but the record may be lacking documentation of the chronicity and frequency that characterize Category I behavior. In addition, evidence is lacking regarding the extent and quality of the prevention program at that level. In other words, these may be students whose aggressive behavior problems, at least in part, may have been occasioned and exacerbated by a previous school environment conducive to those behaviors. Category II students lack the obvious, compelling need characteristics seen in Category I students.

The famous literary detective, Sherlock Holmes, when asked about his procedure for accurately identifying the particulars in a murder case, remarked, "Eliminate all other factors, and the one which remains must be the truth." This bit of wisdom has relevance to the issue of how to go about the process of effectively identifying those students best suited for anger and aggression management skills training. For these students, the "factors" that need to be eliminated are those associated with *resistance to well-designed, universal codes of conduct and disciplinary procedures.* In other words, the critical attribute of students under consideration for anger and aggression management skills training is that they have not responded positively to other procedures.

As noted earlier, collaboratively developed, systematically taught and enforced schoolwide codes of conduct that are linked to well-constructed classroom rules are generally sufficient to meet the behavioral needs of the majority of students. A middle or high school that has not first established this essential foundation is at great risk for the identification of "false positives," those students who appear to need selected or indicated prevention measures but in reality do not. However, in schools in which a high-quality code and its associated classroom extensions are missing or not consistently enforced, it becomes difficult or impossible to discriminate the student who is "behaviorally skilled but predisposed to aggression" from the "truly underskilled." In such cases the school building becomes a setting event that increases the probability of aggression because too many students find that the behavior is reinforced and that there is no evident reason for them to control their anger. Consequently, office referrals for physical and verbal aggression escalate. This situation may lead to the ethically, educationally, and financially undesirable circumstance in which students are mislabeled with anger and aggression problems and provided psychological services they do not need.

Veteran educators know that it is not at all unusual for adolescents to have occasional anger outbursts, even those that are accompanied by physical or verbal aggression. In such cases the code of conduct offers the administrator a range of responses, mildly aversive and educational, and the consequences are applied. This is an example of the "least invasive measure" principle: Lacking evidence to the contrary, a presumption is made that knowledge of the code and the consequences for its breach are sufficient to deter future aggressive behavior. Most students with the usual levels of behavioral skills and impulse control can be expected to respond to those consequences with a marked reduction or elimination of that behavior in the future. It is essential that all schools send an unambiguous message to the students by way of day-to-day school functioning that *fair and competent adult professionals are in charge,* will enforce the rules, and will keep students safe. This understanding allows students who possess the skills to manage their own levels of anger and aggression to do so and more reliably reveals those who cannot.

Category II students are generally known to administrators and pupil services personnel, and they may be on a "high watch" status. Prior to referral for anger and aggression management training, however, less invasive, research-supported behavioral supports (e.g., Sprick, Borgmeier, & Nolet, 2002; Sugai, Horner, & Gresham, 2002) driven by functional behavioral assessments (see Watson & Steege, 2003) should be implemented with high treatment integrity, monitored, and documented.

Many schools utilize a behavior consultation team or student support team staffed by personnel from school psychology, guidance, social work, teaching, and administration to case-manage this effort. A functional behavioral assessment (FBA) first seeks to identify "the relationship between the unique characteristics of the individual and the contextual variables that trigger and reinforce behavior" (Watson & Steege, 2003, p. 5). An effective FBA will develop hypotheses regarding the function of the aggressive behavior within a particular school context (e.g., to obtain peer approval or to escape an aversive verbal compliance demand). Further hypotheses will be offered regarding the antecedent or trigger events that serve to increase the likelihood of the aggression and the subsequent consequences that may be reinforcing and maintaining it. From these data the team will devise a research-supported intervention plan that is designed to (1) reduce or eliminate the antecedent conditions, (2) provide an alternative behavior that serves the same or similar function as the aggression, and/or (3) alter the consequence events that may be reinforcing the aggression. This intervention plan will be implemented with high treatment integrity, monitored, and adjusted as necessary.

The use of the FBA to provide critical intervention planning data cannot be over-emphasized. My experience is that many schools will respond to student aggression by "retrofitting" the student into a preconceived intervention that may be favored by a particular teacher or other school staff member. An educator may remark, "We tried time out and positive social praise, but they didn't work." To which the reply should be: "Did you have any data-based reason to believe they would?" Time out and social praise are reasonable and research-supported behavioral supports, but not as interventions for every student's pattern of aggressive behavior. A well-constructed FBA will assist the intervention team in their efforts to individualize the behavioral supports to the function and contingencies of a particular student's pattern of aggressive behavior, as well as save wasted time and energy.

It is the resistance to well-conceived, correctly implemented behavioral supports embedded in a strong universal prevention structure that serves as the identifying criterion for Category II students. Once that resistance, exhibited in the form of repeated incidents of anger-fueled, aggressive outbursts, has been reliably documented, a referral for skills-training consideration is warranted.

Category III: Need Determined by Individual Assessment

The argument here is that professional resources in the school setting should focus on those students whose behavior demonstrates that they have the highest risk and, consequently, the most need for anger and aggression management skills training. The students subsumed under Categories I and II will make up the overwhelming majority of that group, and in some schools the magnitude of their numbers measured against staff resources will preclude the inclusion of other referrals. Schools should focus limited resources where they will do the greatest good for the greatest number of students and refer others to community mental health recourses.

That said, there is a third category of student whose needs for skills training may also be considered. Some adolescents with no documented history of anger or aggression in the school setting may suddenly encounter a transient period of personal stress or turmoil that calls for professional intervention. These stressors may include family, relationship, academic, or other developmentally related problems that have overwhelmed the individual's ability to cope. Category III students have typically demonstrated adaptive behavior in school, and their somewhat sudden entrance into aggressive behavior patterns late in their school experience may surprise school officials.

- A basketball player is suddenly benched for repeated aggressive outbursts on the court.
- A sophomore with no substantive discipline record receives his or her second office referral in a week for threatening behavior.
- A previously mild-mannered student suddenly trashes the chemistry lab.
- A seventh-grade honor student angrily threatens to kill his English teacher.

Because of the sudden-onset nature of the problem behavior, the inclusion of Category III students in a skills-training intervention must come only following a comprehensive psychological assessment by the school psychologist or other qualified mental health professional. The possibility of co-occuring clinical conditions, such as depression, anxiety, or delayed reaction to trauma, must be considered carefully. In such cases the school professional must have a clear understanding of the hierarchical nature of the presenting problems and address treatment priorities accordingly. For instance, it may well be that a particular student would benefit from learning a repertoire of anger coping skills but that therapy to address depression will take precedence in the treatment hierarchy in this case. For students with co-occurring mental health concerns, the value of establishing solid, collaborative relationships with community mental health professionals cannot be overstated.

Summary

The decision to remove adolescents from a portion of their normal curricular schedule and place them in an anger and aggression skills management training group should be acted on only with the greatest of care and attention to valid and reliable sources of information. Secondary school personnel need to be thoroughly informed regarding the behavior documented in historical education records of incoming students, as such information may be usefully predictive of future behavior. Additionally, the value that comes from observing a student's adjustment to a well-operationalized primary prevention structure and the added component of data-driven positive behavioral supports can be of significant decision-making importance. Finally, school personnel need to be cognizant that student anger and aggression may be symptoms of underlying mental health concerns. Assuring that these possible concerns are not overlooked in the zeal to provide an intervention for the highly salient behavior is a professional and ethical obligation of the school.

PREINTERVENTION ASSESSMENT

When a well-screened student is identified as someone who may benefit from anger and aggression management skills, the group leaders need to undertake a pre-intervention assessment. The essential questions that this assessment should seek to answer include:

1. What is the current frequency of the student's aggressive behavior in the school?
2. Under what conditions and locations and in whose presence is the aggression most likely to occur? Least likely?
3. What is the hypothesized function or purpose of the aggression for the student?
4. Which consequences seem to reinforce the aggression and which seem to reduce it?
5. How great a part does poorly controlled anger play in the aggressive behavior?

When the preintervention assessment is complete, the group leaders should have a preliminary answer to the question: What does this student need to know and be able to do in the general school setting to reduce or eliminate further aggressive behavior? The following are essential components.

Record Review

Once a referral for anger and aggression management training has been made, it is now up to the anger and aggression management group leaders (hereinafter referred to as "trainers") to decide on the nature and extent of further assessment procedures. If students have been identified through the processes described in Categories I and II, then the trainers should have a wealth of critical information already available to them. For these students it is typically no longer a question of whether or not the intervention is warranted, because that issue has been decided by previous and continuing intervention efforts. The student has either demonstrated a compelling, ongoing need for skills-training support reflected in data from previous levels of schooling

(Category I) or the student has exhausted less intrusive schoolwide and classroom behavioral supports in the current environment (Category II). In the course of these efforts, considerable data will have been accumulated. Training group leaders need to use these data to help assess the continuing education and skill needs of the individual students referred for the group (see Appendix B: "Intervention Record Review").

In the student's office, cumulative, and intervention records:

- Examine for possible patterns or similarities in office discipline referrals. Are incidents of anger or aggression related more to interactions with adults or with peers? Do they have a temporal pattern, for example, mostly afternoons or mostly Fridays? Are there particular setting events of concern, such as the lunchroom, math classes, the shop area, the physical education facilities, or other physical settings, that seem to occasion high levels of problem behavior? Is a substantial percentage of the office referrals from only one or two adults, indicating a possible training need focused on managing those future interactions?

- Scrutinize the types and effectiveness of previous schoolwide and classroom behavioral supports. Have some of them demonstrated effectiveness, and do they deserve to be maintained or reinstated? What does the relative success or failure of these supports say about the skill level of this student? For example, the previous success or failure of a voluntary "cool down" room may provide information about the student's ability to self-monitor anger levels.

- Examine the record for previous counseling or skills-training efforts within the recent past. With appropriate releases of information, arrange a conference with one of the former group leaders to discuss the student's participation, behavior management strategies, and skill level at termination.

- Become fully aware of co-occurring academic problems and deficiencies. What are the student's historical academic strengths and weaknesses? What academic supports are currently in place, and are they proving effective? What data are available from "high stakes" or other group testing? What is the high school student's units-to-graduation status? The need for group leaders to monitor academic progress and behavior and to work collaboratively with teachers cannot be overemphasized.

Student Interview

For the trainers, the initial interview is an opportunity to "fill in some gaps" left by the examination of the record and to put a human face on the referred student. The interviewer needs to remain cognizant of the fact that although this is a data-gathering encounter, it may also be an opportunity to start the seeds of the therapeutic relationship to come. Consequently, a supportive, interested, and nonjudgmental attitude is preferable to a more detached, purely assessment-oriented style. My experience is that friendliness and common respect go a long way with many youths who may not be used to it from the adults in their lives. A much more in-depth treatment of the many complexities associated with the interviewing of adolescents in general may be found in Sattler (1997, 2002).

An individual, pretreatment interview with the adolescent referred for anger and aggression management training should include the following assessment elements (see Appendix C: "Adolescent Interview"):

1. *The student's understanding of the problem behavior, including origins and current status.* For many youths with serious aggressive behavior difficulties, speaking with adults in the school about their behavior may be a somewhat common event, and they will demonstrate commendable insight into their histories and personal struggles. As noted earlier, however, cognitive distortions, including misattribution of intent, are characteristic of many youths with reactive aggression. The interviewer should expect to find some students denying responsibility for much of the behavior of which they are accused. In such cases the interviewer needs to consider the possibility that the student may honestly believe that he or she is being victimized by more aggressive individuals and that that is the "explanation" for all of the serious disciplinary problems. Alternative considerations are that the student is lying in an effort to make this irritating experience go away or is engaging in some combination of both distortion and untruthfulness. The interview situation is not the forum wherein to disentangle these hypotheses but merely to acquire data for later use.

2. *The student's understanding of current and previous efforts to address the problem.* Most adolescents of average intellectual functioning are mature enough to be cognizant of what the adults around them are trying to do to change their behavior. In this aspect of the interview, the interviewer wants to gauge the level of that insight and solicit from the student an opinion about the relative success of these efforts. For example, why did the point system fail to prevent additional aggressive episodes, or why was the "cool down" room so useful? The interviewer also needs to gather insight into the student's sense of the efficacy of his or her own self-control strategies. Many students will assert that they can control their anger and aggression "when I want to." Given the behavioral record, this leads to the hypotheses that they either have a distorted sense of their own ability to control their aggressive responses or are poor judges of the environmental cues that indicate the need. Both hypotheses point to training needs.

3. *The student's willingness to participate in the skills-training group.* Mental health professionals in the school setting need to consider the student's personal opinion, along with other factors, when considering an individual for enrollment in a skills-training group.

Legally in the school setting, informed consent for psychological services rests with the parents of a minor child. However, the practitioner is obligated ethically to respect the dignity, autonomy, and self-determination of the student/client. The decision to allow a student/client the opportunity to choose (or refuse) psychological treatment or intervention may involve the consideration of a number of factors, including law, ethical issues (self-determination versus welfare of the client), the pupil's competence to make choices, and the likely consequence of affording choices. . . . (Jacob & Hartshorne, 2003, p. 188)

Before the close of the interview, the interviewer should talk to the student about the skills-training group for which he or she is being considered. In addition where legally mandated, the student should be informed that a parental consent letter will be forthcoming. In my experience it is an extremely rare circumstance in which the student will decline to attend the first session, if only for the opportunity to get out of a class. It is during that upcoming first session that a more expansive discussion of the training particulars is offered, and the student should be assured that he or she may choose to refuse participation at that time.

Teacher/Administrator Interview

The group leaders should select for interview those adults who have regular contact with the referred student and who can offer insight into the possible causes and contingencies of the aggressive behavior. The information acquired from these interviews should not only cover the problem behaviors and environments but also those conditions under which the student seems to regularly function in a more adaptive, less aggressive manner. Along with selected classroom teachers, the administrator or dean who has the most frequent contact with the student for disciplinary reasons should be interviewed. A sample interview form is included in Appendix D, "Brief Problem Assessment Interview."

Authentic Data

What are the current "official" indicators of problem behavior in this particular school setting? The paper trail providing the answer to this question makes up what is known as authentic data. During the preintervention period, it is essential for group leaders to catalogue these data as indicators of the need for an additional intervention, as well as a potential "clinical baseline" from which to gauge intervention progress. This record can include (1) the accumulated number of office referrals for anger-related behavioral difficulties, (2) classroom detention referrals, (3) school absentee and classroom tardy slips, and (4) selected academic progress indicators. In addition, any other schoolwide or classroom-level measure of behavior, positive or negative, that can reasonably be expected to be affected by improved self-control may be included.

A procedure should be devised so that information from the selected data sources can be monitored, acquired, and maintained in graphical form by the trainers throughout the intervention and postintervention periods. It is recommended that trainers allow the students to self-monitor their own progress. One of my interns recently developed a system in which the main office staff provided her with discipline, attendance, and tardy records on a weekly basis and she had each group member enter his or her own data into a spreadsheet program prior to the start of the session. Line graphs were printed out on a regular basis. A more low-tech format utilizing a sheet of poster board and a permanent marker would work equally well. These data can assist the group leaders in keeping their focus on the who, what, and where issues that are actually happening with the students so as to better link the training skills to actual persons and events in school.

If the school does not keep the kind of official record that the trainers believe to be the best monitor of training progress, then it is incumbent on them to develop and establish one that is more applicable. As an example, the "Classroom Progress Monitoring Reportø (Appendix E) provides a sample weekly classroom monitoring form for teachers to complete and return to the group leaders. My experience is that the complexity of the monitoring form is inversely proportional to the likelihood of its being completed regularly: Keep it simple. Trainers utilizing a form such as this should be aware that a recent, highly salient negative event can cause a teacher to skew weekly averages lower. Encourage them to think broadly across the week.

Authentic data that monitor what is *actually* occurring in the school setting can provide an important counterbalance to what some individuals *believe* to be occurring. High-profile, highly externalizing, and aggressive middle or high school students are simply not going to make "silver bullet" changes because they enter a skills-training group. In fact, to the casual observer (e.g., a teacher or administrator), it may appear that there is no change at all. Yet a student who had 20 and 23 office referrals in the 2 months prior to the start of the group and now is averaging 14 per month at group's end has shown clear progress. It may take the visual presentation of these data to all parties to help convince them of both the value of the intervention and the effort of the student. No one wants an effective intervention to be discarded because it did not "appear" to be effective.

Individual Psychometric Inventories

Individual psychometric data are essential for researchers examining the effects of a particular intervention on a set of variables, and this is no less true for anger and aggression interventions than it is for other areas of school concern. For example, research on three of the most widely respected anger interventions, the Art of Self-Control (Feindler, Marriott, & Iwata, 1984; Feindler, Ecton, Kingsley, & Dubey, 1986), the Anger Coping Program (Lochman & Curry, 1986; Lochman & Lampron, 1986), and Aggression Replacement Training (Goldstein et al., 1986, 1998) utilized psychometric self-, teacher-, and parent-report data to clarify effects and demonstrate

potential usefulness. This level of research is an important prerequisite to establishing the potential usefulness of an intervention for practitioners in an applied setting.

School psychologists and counselors in the educational setting are typically less interested in these "paper" effects and substantially more interested in observable behavior change. Trainers and their supervisors are much more concerned about altering behavior in the building than they are about seeing change on an anger inventory. Consequently, the decision to gather individual assessment data from published scales and inventories should be driven by the existence of hypotheses concerning the problem behavior that have not been answered by other means. For young children still at the elementary level, individual psychometric assessment data acquired through self-report or teacher inventories are very useful in the effort to better understand the structure and function of the problematic behavior (see Larson & Lochman, 2002). However, by the start of middle or high school, educators often have acquired a useful understanding of whether a particular student's aggression is a function of poorly controlled emotional arousal, a significant deficit in problem-solving skills, proactive-type "bully" aggression, or some combination of all three. In such instances the need for additional psychometric evidence to corroborate substantial existing observational and archival school data is often unnecessary.

Many practitioners are interested in gathering teacher- or self-report data to enhance those obtained through observation, interview, and record review. Most school psychologists are familiar with the Behavior Assessment System for Children (BASC; Reynolds & Kamphaus, 1992) and Child Behavior Checklist (CBCL; Achenbach, 1991). These two well-designed and psychometrically sound checklists can provide insight into the teacher's perception of the student along numerous externalizing subscales. In my experience, however, I have found broadband teacher rating scales such as these to be insensitive to behavior change, even in the face of compelling authentic school behavioral data to the contrary.

Two of the most widely used research and clinical instruments to assess self-reported anger and aggressive behavior in young persons are the Children's Inventory of Anger (ChIA; Nelson & Finch, 2000) and the State–Trait Anger Inventory—2 (STAXI-2; Spielberger, 1999). The ChIA is a self-report measure for ages 6 through 16 that yields subtest scores in the factors of Frustration, Physical Aggression, Peer Relationships, and Authority Relations. The format is a 39-item Likert-type scale that presents the respondents with a simple scenario (e.g., "Someone takes your bike without your permission") and provides a continuum of possible anger response levels from "not at all" to "furious." Although the authors suggest an age range up to 16, the inventory scenarios are clearly most relevant to the younger end of the age range. The STAXI-2 (Spielberger, 1999) is a 57-item self-report scale for individuals ages 16 to adult. The inventory examines "state anger" (Feeling Angry, Feel Like Expressing Anger Verbally, Feel Like Expressing Anger Physically), "trait anger" (Angry Temperament, Angry Reaction), and five additional subscales. An Anger

Expression Index is yielded that provides an overall measure of total anger expression. This instrument and its first-edition predecessor have been a staple in the adult anger assessment literature for many years, but the age range for school use is confining, and the instrument's sixth-grade reading level can prove problematic for some students.

A promising addition to the field that has greater relevance to school personnel is currently undergoing research trials both in the United States and abroad. The Multidimensional School Anger Inventory (MSAI; Smith, Furlong, Bates, & Laughlin, 1998) is an attempt to measure how anger manifests itself in the school setting.

> The MSAI is based on a three-component model of the global anger process that involves an emotional–affective component, a cognitive hostility–cynicism component, and a behavioral–expressive component. Alpha coefficients are .86 for Anger Experience, .80 for Hostility, .82 for Destructive Expression, and .68 for Positive Coping. Test–retest reliabilities over a six-month period ranged from .56 to .62 for the four subscales. (M. J. Furlong, personal communication, January 26, 2004)

The current research version of the MSAI has been included as Appendix F and is available for practitioner use as an added data-gathering resource and, for those engaging in applied research, as a supplementary measure of program treatment effects. Interested individuals should visit *www.education.ucsb.edu/c4sbyd* for a user's manual and ongoing access to the latest information and validity studies of this instrument. For those practitioners interested in other psychometric measures to further their understanding of the students or demonstrate treatment effects for an applied research effort, useful reviews of current measures may be found in Feindler and Baker (2001) and Furlong and Smith (1994).

SUMMARY

Training students in anger and aggression management skills, whether accomplished in a small-group format or individual treatment, is a labor-intensive and time-consuming endeavor that forces highly skilled professionals to put aside some of their other important duties and responsibilities for the duration. In addition, the students who are participating in this training are labeled with anger and aggression problems and may be taken out of academic classes or other important educational activities in order to take part. Consequently, the decisions associated with this undertaking must be approached with attention to valid and reliable screening and identification procedures. Middle and high schools must establish collaborative information-sharing relationships with their feeder schools so that the needs of entering students with problem behavior can be better understood and addressed without undue delay. The potential for misidentification is reduced when the school has an effective schoolwide prevention and discipline program, teachers skilled in classroom management strategies, and pupil services personnel skilled in FBA and positive behavioral supports. Finally, the preintervention assessment of referred students should seek to acquire as much information as reasonably possible regarding environmental and student variables that contribute to the problem behavior.

CHAPTER 5

◆ ◆ ◆

Getting Started with Anger and Aggression Management Skills Training

◆

With the potential group members identified and the preintervention assessment complete, it is time to start preparations for the first meeting. Careful attention to these preparatory tasks will allow the group to run as efficiently and effectively as possible and prevent potential problems down the line.

INFORMED PARENTAL CONSENT

As noted in Chapter 4, parents are responsible for consenting to psychological services for their minor children (Jacob & Hartshorne, 2003). The cognitive-behavioral orientation of the skills training that is advocated and described in this book undeniably constitutes "psychological services," regardless of which license or certification its group leaders hold. A guidance counselor or a school social worker who is utilizing behavioral and cognitive therapeutic methods to alter the thinking and behavior of a minor student is providing psychological treatment, and informed parental consent is needed. For school psychologists, the requirement to obtain parental consent prior to engaging in any intervention is made clear almost from their first day in graduate school. For guidance counselors, whose professional counseling activities are often subsumed under what is referred to as "ordinary schooling," consent issues may be less a part of their normal experience. All school mental health professionals are encouraged to consult a recognized text that addresses these and related issues (e.g., Jacob & Hartshorne, 2003) and to confer with their local legal authority regarding individual state laws and customary procedures.

I often present my graduate students with this scenario:

"Imagine that you are the parent of a 12-year-old seventh-grade student who announces one night at dinner, 'I didn't have to take my English test today because I had Anger Problem group.' If that was the first time that you as a parent ever heard the term 'anger problem group' in association with your child, might it give you cause for concern? Who said you have an *anger problem*? What *group*? You missed *English*?"

Granted, if the identification process has been followed as described in Chapter 4, there is a high likelihood that the parent is well aware that their child has been experiencing behavioral problems in school and may be happy for the service, but that does not negate the need for consent. In my experience the great majority of parents fall somewhere between ambivalent and delighted at the prospect of this intervention, and over my two decades of direct service and supervision, I can count on one hand the numbers who have declined consent. Sample parental consent letters, in English and in Spanish, are included in Appendix G.

The single greatest obstacle in this process is the actual transmission of the consent form to the home and back. In theory, the form is handed to the student to take home, have signed, and promptly return to the school. Most of us who work with adolescents (or have one of our own) are well aware that many items of timely importance are placed into "the Black Hole of the book bag" and, defying some principle of physics, never seen again. After the first or second attempt, group leaders should consider the following in approximately this order:

- Place a phone call to the parents, suggesting that they ask their child for it.
- Provide a monetary or other incentive to the student for its return, watching for forgeries.
- Mail the form to the parent with a self-addressed stamped return envelope and follow up with a phone call.
- Mail the form via certified mail that requires a signed receipt.
- Visit the parent at home and obtain the signature.

Providing mental health services in the school to minor students without parental consent is a practice fraught with legal and ethical risk, yet questions regarding the need for older adolescents to obtain parental consent frequently arise among mental health professionals in the high school setting. In such instances informed, professional judgment must prevail. For instance, if a mentally competent 16- or 17-year-old student expressly desires to participate in the group and offers a compelling reason why contact with the parents would be dangerous or inappropriate (e.g., the potential for abuse or clear questions about the mental capacity of the parent to provide informed consent), are group leaders within legal or ethical boundaries to allow the student to participate? As noted earlier, it is important that school personnel understand the guiding legal authority and the professional ethics that govern decision making about such practices in their local jurisdiction and profession. The school system's legal counsel or the local district attorney can serve as a resource to help clarify the legal aspects of this issue. In addition, posing the question to a state ethics board can provide practitioners with useful guidance and supporting documentation for their future decision making.

GENERALIZATION ISSUES: AVOID "TRAIN AND HOPE"

Perhaps the greatest challenge for trainers and the students they work with is generalizing skills to the authentic environment of the school building. As Meichenbaum (2001) noted: "The training and treatment literature are replete with examples of intervention programs that sound encouraging, but they often fail to evidence generalization or transfer across settings, across response domains, and over time" (p. 334). Practitioners and their student clients can work hard in the group room week after week, but if there is no systematic plan for generalization, all that time and effort may be for naught. Worse yet, extending effort in therapy only to experience no subsequent "real life" improvement may permanently sour a young person on the value of seeking therapeutic support in the future. Utilizing generalization procedures and activities in the skills-training experience itself is discussed later, but before the group even has its first session, what can the trainers do to assist the transfer of skills to the general school environment? The answer to this lies in maximizing the potential generalization influence of other adults in the school setting.

The student's upcoming participation in a skills-training group to address anger and aggression control cannot be approached with the same level of respect for personal privacy that therapists would assure for most other presenting concerns. This is due in part to the already highly visible, externalizing nature of the behavior in question and the need for knowledgeable adults in the general setting to assist in the transfer of training. With many other, more internalizing-type concerns, such as mild depression or adolescent adjustment problems, the school psychologist or counselor may see less of a need to involve other school professionals outside of the actual therapy situation. However, aggressive behavior that has been unresponsive to an array of focused disciplinary measures and behavioral supports demands that others become actively involved to support the training. Consequently, selected teachers and administrators should be identified as generalization supports. These individuals should be made aware that a particular student will be engaging in skills training to manage anger and aggression and enlisted to provide support for the student's efforts to enact newly acquired skills in the authentic setting.

In addition, the students themselves should be made aware of who the generalization-support adults in the school are and why they were chosen. For example:

"Gerald, in order to help and support you to make the changes we have discussed, we have obtained the assistance of Mr. Conrad, the assistant principal, Ms. Johnson, your English teacher, and Ms. Carter, the lunchroom duty teacher. They have volunteered to provide you with whatever support they can to help you. This might include privately pointing out to you when you are doing a good job with your new skills or giving you feedback after a slip-up. I know that the end of the day has been a difficult time for you, so that is why I asked Ms. Johnson, your seventh-period teacher, to help. We both know the lunchroom has been hard for you to handle some days, and, of course, you and Mr. Conrad are good friends, so I couldn't leave him out. I will be meeting with them regularly for feedback on how things are going. Do you have any problems with my selections, or is there an additional person you would like me to ask as well?"

A cautionary note: The students' rights to confidentiality in the therapeutic relationship must be maintained as prescribed by governing ethical codes and guiding legal authorities. Other adults are enlisted as supports for transfer of training only, and their need to know the particulars of what is said in the confines of the therapy situation is *limited strictly to that which is necessary to carry out those responsibilities and no more.* If the need arises for the group leaders to reveal more than general training progress and recommendations for support behaviors to the identified adults, then the student should be informed of what will be revealed and for what purpose. For instance, a group leader may determine that a student's uncharacteristically furious anger at his or her parent, expressed in the group meeting, may increase the likelihood of anger control problems later in the day. In such a situation the group leader should speak privately with the student and inform him or her of the reason and extent of any communication with other adults regarding that issue. For example, "I'm going to let your support people know that you're feeling pretty angry today. I won't mention anything about home, just that you are having a tough day. Is there something I can ask them to do that might help?"

Teachers and Administrators as Generalization Supports

Teachers at the middle and, particularly, the high school level are less able than their elementary-level counterparts to commit large amounts time and energy to the extraordinary needs of one or two students. In my experience, this is due much more to time constraints dictated by the large number of students they see daily than it is by their willingness to help. In general, I have found secondary-level teachers very willing to do what they can within the confines of their responsibilities to their many other students. If the trainers are sensitive to the teachers' needs, the likelihood of an effective collaborative relationship is enhanced.

Generalization support for this intervention demands little in the way of additional duties for the identified individuals. They are being asked only to observe the student in the context of their relationship with him or her (e.g., classroom, shop, gymnasium, duty area) and, when feasible, offer behavioral feedback and positive support for change efforts (see Appendix H, "Guidelines for Generalization Support Persons"). Regular, brief, and informal meetings with the group leaders are also required.

When selecting a teacher to function as a generalization-support person, adhering to as many of the following guidelines as possible is recommended:

- Choose a teacher who may already have a positive relationship with the student.
- Choose a teacher who interacts with the student in a context or time of day that has been historically problematic.
- With students in special education, prefer general education teachers over special education teachers, as there is an expectation that the latter already have supportive relationships with their students.
- Choose a teacher with high status among the general student body and thus, perhaps, high status also with the identified student.
- Many middle schools have a team or house structure, with a common preparatory period for discussing students. If the entire team volunteers, group leaders should take them up on it, but designate a principal liaison.

Group leaders should always select one administrator as a generalization support person. As a useful rule of thumb, when a choice is available, select the administrator who is most visible around the school and thus most likely to have regular contact with the student. Previous relationships are also important in this selection. Students with high levels of problematic behavior may have soured their relationship with the administrator responsible for discipline, so care must be taken on this count. If the selection is satisfactory to both the student and the adult, that administrator can be a very influential support. On the other hand, if one or both are unwilling or unable to alter their negative feelings, identifying that person as a generalization support may be unwise. My experience on this issue is that most administrators are professional enough to adjust their roles in the direction of support when possible and that most students are willing to take a cautionary "wait and see" position before dismissing the possibility altogether.

WHAT ABOUT GIRLS?

In the late 1980s, when I was with the Milwaukee Public Schools' violence prevention program, our team typically started our work in a secondary-level building by meeting with the principal to discuss the plan. In our early naiveté, we believed that this administrator would be delighted that we intended to identify the most aggressive, behaviorally problematic boys and begin skills-training groups with them. Virtually to a person, that plan was met with some plaintive variation of, "But what about the *girls*?" In Milwaukee at that time, the boys' aggression was grabbing the newspaper headlines, but it was the girls who were making teachers' and administrators' lives miserable.

Understanding girls' anger and aggression has come a long way since that time. The seminal work of Nikki Crick and colleagues on relational aggression (e.g., Crick, 1996, 1997; Crick & Bigbee, 1998; Crick & Grotpeter, 1995; Crick et al., 2001; Crick & Werner, 1998) and groundbreaking insights into physically aggressive girls (e.g., Adams, 1992; Pepler & Sedighdeilami, 1998; Pepler & Craig, 1999) have added considerably to our understanding. Yet with respect to similar research with boys, to date there have been very few empirically supported differential intervention strategies developed for aggressive girls in the school context. This is clearly a serious gap in the literature that demands attention.

A promising, gender-specific intervention for aggressive girls in the 5- to 12-year-old range is currently being implemented and studied in Canada. The Earlscourt Girls Connection (Walsh, Pepler, & Levine, 2002) uses a developmental model of risk and protective factors to inform the intervention in three primary areas: individual behaviors, primary relationship contexts (including parent–child and family), and secondary contexts (including school and community). Parent training procedures assist parents in obtaining skills in monitoring behavior, effective use of reinforcements and aversive consequences, and improved interpersonal communication. The child-focused intervention is informed by the sociocognitive information processing deficits of aggressive children and youth (e.g., Crick & Dodge, 1994) and has anger management and social-problem-solving components. Preliminary analysis of 98 girls who completed the program was promising, indicating reductions in parent-reported incidences of aggression and improved relationships with both teachers and parents at both 6- and 12-month follow-ups (Pepler et al., in press).

Many of the same factors that put adolescent boys at risk for aggressive behavior in school appear to operate also for girls (Pepler & Sedighdeilami, 1998). Rejection by the prosocial peer group and affiliation with antisocial peers, low connectedness to the school, and a history of school-context aggressive behavior are risk factors for both girls and boys as they enter middle or high school. Consequently, the screening and identification procedures for girls should follow those for boys (see Chapter 4). In addition, school personnel should be cognizant of the findings that (1) girls who have been physically or sexually abused in the home have an increased risk for physically aggressive behavior (Pepler & Sedighdeilami, 1998); (2) verbal aggression and intimidation by girls in the elementary school setting may be a predictor of physical aggression in the secondary school setting (Leschied, Cummings, Van Brunschot, Cunningham, & Saunders, 2000), and (3) with the onset of puberty, girls are as much as three times more likely than boys to experience depression, which, in association with other factors, can increase the probability of aggressive behavior (Lescheid et al., 2000).

The procedures contained in the anger management program discussed in this volume can be implemented in the treatment of girls' aggressive school-context behavior with the addition of the following:

1. The group experience should allow for evident victimization issues to be openly addressed, facilitated by trainers who have the requisite skill and training in these issues.
2. The focused use of situation-specific, adaptive aggression as a self-protection measure in the context of abuse should be discussed and the possibility of professional training assessed and implemented as needed.
3. The addition of a further social-skills component (e.g., Goldstein & McGinnis, 2000) and additional emphasis on assertiveness training should be considered.
4. The possibility of co-occurring depression, particularly among middle school girls, should be carefully examined and appropriate treatment provided.

Individuals interested in further insights into the needs of aggressive adolescent girls may find the following useful: *Beyond Appearance: A New Look at Adolescent Girls* (Johnson, Roberts, & Worell, 1999); *Social Aggression Among Girls* (Underwood, 2003); and *The Development and Treatment of Girlhood Aggression* (Pepler, Madsen, Webster, & Levine, 2004).

DEVELOPING A GROUP BEHAVIOR MANAGEMENT AND INCENTIVE STRATEGY

When working with younger students with anger and aggression control problems in the elementary school setting, a carefully constructed and strict behavior management plan is essential (Larson & Lochman, 2002). As students get older and developmentally predictable silliness, impulsivity, and physical activity start to abate, the need for such highly structured in-group management plans to keep undesirable behavior under control becomes less critical. (Trainers who are targeting particularly immature middle school students may want to consult Larson and Lochman, 2002, for a suggested strategy.) This does not obviate the need for a behavior management strategy with secondary-level students; it merely changes the target of the behavior.

Woody Allen is reported to have quipped that "Eighty percent of life is just showing up." Influencing the referred adolescents to regularly "show up" at the designated time and place is one of the first great goals of an effective behavior management plan. With elementary-level students, the group leaders have considerable control over this basic issue. This typically involves little more than walking to the classroom, gathering them up, and escorting them back to the group room. However, there is no greater way to ensure resistance in an adolescent than for a school psychologist to appear at the door of a ninth-grade classroom and signal for the student to come along. The personal discomfort occasioned by the journey past the desks of his or her commenting peers is not something that will soon be forgiven.

Therapy with voluntary and "other than voluntary" students in the school setting requires that the professional take into account the student's motivation to participate. Most mental health workers in the secondary schools are very familiar with that subset of students who initiate contact with the professional because they are seeking relief from intrapersonal or interpersonal concerns. Accompanying this contact is some level of within-client motivation to keep appointments and follow through with therapy recommendations, at least initially. In contrast, it is important to remember that the adolescents who will be participating in the anger and aggression management skills group are highly unlikely to be self-referrals and that, as a result, their level of internal motivation to relieve personal discomfort is most often slight or absent altogether. The initial interview may have stimulated enough curiosity for the group members to show up for the first meeting, and this will provide an opportunity for a well-planned intellectual rationale to be offered in favor of continuance. However, I have left enough first sessions absolutely convinced that I "had them," only to be looking at empty chairs the next week, to have gained a much more humble assessment of the power of oral persuasion. External incentives and a structured reminder–transition process to bolster the probability that the adolescent will even show up for the second meeting are essential.

The following suggestions are based on my experience and that of many colleagues and interns who have implemented group treatment for anger and aggression management in the middle and high schools. Each school will have its own idiosyncratic procedures and potential barriers within which trainers must operate.

Reminder–Transition

1. If possible, program incoming high-risk students with a common study hall or common academic team to facilitate easier accessibility.

2. Never leave the responsibility to remember the next meeting time to the students alone. Reminder cards, notes in daily planners, and prewritten hall passes help but are generally insufficient even if they do not become lost.

3. Contact the teacher who will be excusing the student for group on the day of the meeting, either in person or with a hall pass in his or her mail box.

4. Consider laminated hall passes with the student's name and the time and room location of the group. Collect them at the end of each session and redistribute them to the excusing teacher the following week.

5. Consider an announcement over the public address system. For example, "Attention members of the Think First organization: The weekly meeting will be held today during fifth period." At one school the students asked to be summoned by name. Leave this decision up to the group members.

6. To avoid delays and unnecessary interpersonal hassles between adults and group members, provide hall aides and staff members on hall duty with a written list of the names of students who will be in transition to the group room.

Incentives

1. A critical incentive with young people is an agreeable experience. The trainers increase cooperation to the degree that they treat the group members with respect, understanding, and empathy for their difficult circumstances. It is important to take the perspective that these students have ended up in the group in large measure because of the effects of personal and environmental risk factors over which they may have had no control or influence (what one of my interns referred to as the "There but for the grace of God . . . " insight). Providing a unique context that does not include blame, judgment, or retribution on the one hand or manufactured pity on the other can be a rewarding experience for many historically problematic adolescents.

2. The use of tangible reinforcers to influence attendance and behavioral cooperation has been demonstrated over time to be useful. Trainers should acquire a monetary budget from the school or another granting source sufficient to purchase potentially reinforcing small-ticket merchandise. Items such as fast food and movie coupons have been found to be effective, but input from group members should be solicited. A system that allows group members to earn points for attendance and other designated behaviors that can be exchanged for the reinforcers should be designed ahead of time.

3. Behaviors that earn points can include attendance, completion of out-of-group behavioral tasks, participation and peer support in the group, and other behaviors that the group leaders desire to increase in frequency. Points for desirable behaviors should be maintained by the group leaders in a manner easily reviewed by the group members.

4. Consider allowing the group members to have input into the "cost" of the various reinforcers. For instance, the group may agree that a fast-food coupon may be "purchased" for 10 points but that the movie coupon requires 25 points. Group leaders should agree on contingencies that will allow for exchanges approximately every third meeting.

5. Consider securing a "community partner" who will assist with funds for reinforcers. Some businesses are more open to sponsoring specific projects in the school than to contributing to a more general fund, and, once on board, they appreciate regular updates regarding how their contributions are helping. As a suggestion, group leaders may want to approach the local association that represents law enforcement in their community for support.

6. Consider an "academic supplies grab bag" as an attendance reinforcer. Have a container filled with pencils, pens, loose-leaf paper, and other consumables from which group members can restock their own needs at the conclusion of each session.

7. "The way to an adolescent's brain is though his stomach" is an adage worth remembering. A candy bar or other small snack at the conclusion of the group can add immeasurably to the general agreeableness of the experience. I highly recommend it. It is worthwhile to survey group members' preferences and dietary restrictions before purchasing in bulk, however. Additionally, this instance is not the time to take a personal stand against junk food in young people's diet, but rather a time to use every weapon at one's disposal.

THINK FIRST: RATIONALE AND REVIEW OF THE RESEARCH

The remainder of this book discusses the implementation of a skills-training intervention titled Think First: Anger and Aggression Management for Secondary-Level Students. This intervention was developed initially by my friend and colleague, Judith A. McBride, PhD, and me from Feindler and Ecton's (1986) pioneering adolescent anger program, "The Art of Self-Control." Think First represents an effort to bring well-established cognitive-behavioral techniques and procedures in manualized form to the problem of aggressive behavior in the school setting.

The initial study on Think First was accomplished as a part of my doctoral dissertation at Marquette University in Milwaukee. In 1988, a series of highly publicized fighting incidents at a number of the city's high schools had motivated the Milwaukee Public Schools' Board of School Directors to create the violence reduction program. I was one of two individuals assigned to that program, and one of our first responsibilities was to address the violence in the high schools. Along with the implementation of a classroom-level violence prevention curriculum, our approach was to locate an existing anger management intervention and adapt it for use in the schools. Our review turned up a group anger control program that had been developed and studied by Eva Feindler and her colleagues (Feindler et al., 1986; Feindler et al., 1984) and published as a session-by-session program (Feindler & Ecton, 1986).

Following the conclusion of four pilot anger control groups completed during the spring semester of 1989, the decision was made to restructure Feindler and Ecton's (1986) program to take better advantage of the training potentials contained in the school environment. What had become clear to us was that we were simply retrofitting a clinical intervention into the educational setting. The adolescents we were seeing in the groups might just as well have been receiving the same intervention in a community agency for all the attention that was paid to their actual school issues. These youths were supremely disinterested in anything school related and wanted only to address what they believed to be their most vital concerns—what happened at a house party over the weekend, who pulled a gun on whom Tuesday night, what gang is moving into what neighborhood, and so on. Importantly, they were resistant to our efforts to train them in anger control procedures and regularly scoffed at what they perceived to be our naiveté about the skills needed for street survival. Our poor outcome measures reflected these problems.

School Focus

During the summer of 1989, Judith McBride and I restructured the intervention and made a series of supporting videos to be used as behavioral models. Our goal was to create a more school-friendly intervention that maximized the expertise of the trainers, minimized their weaknesses, and offered greater potential for student change. To do this, we pulled the entire focus of the skills training back into the school setting. No longer would community problems be the center of discussion and training; in effect, we banned them from the intervention. Our rationale for this decision was twofold: (1) School-based professionals had greater potential for high credibility regarding issues of "hallway survival" than "street survival," and (2) the students were referred for school-based problems, and those were serious enough to demand exclusive concentration.

In making this decision, we were not ignorant of the often reciprocal nature of community and school behavior problems. On the contrary, our sensitivity to the effects of a violent community on the problems in its schools was heightened. However, effecting change among adolescents with serious externalizing behavior is a daunting challenge under any circumstances. Limiting the context to the area of greatest trainer influence allowed for a more focused effort and potentially improved student outcomes. In effect, one of our goals was to train the students to enter the building and alter their street-survival skills to meet the demands for success in the school environment.

Research Review

Think First was implemented for study in the fall of 1989 at a Milwaukee central city middle school (see Larson, 1991; 1992). Participants were drawn from an existing program for at-risk students. Thirteen male and nine female students received the Think First training, whereas a control group consisting of nine male and six female students were in a discussion-only condition. In the experimental group, 14 students identified themselves as black, and 8 identified themselves as white. In the control group, the racial split was 10 and 5, respectively. The groups met on a weekly basis for 10 weeks. Data were gathered through psychometric measures that examined self-reported anger expression, attitudes toward criminal behavior, and teacher assessment of aggressive behavior. Additional data were maintained on office referrals for disruptive or aggressive behavior. At the conclusion of the treatment, a repeated-measures ANOVA performed on the psychometric variables found no interaction between the treatment condition and time of measurement. However, with regard to the number of office referrals for disruptive or aggressive behavior, the Think First group showed a .18 decrease per student from baseline to follow-up, and the control group students showed a .80 increase per student for the same time period, a difference that was statistically significant.

Nickerson (2003) examined the effects of the Think First program on four ninth- and tenth-grade classrooms at a large, ethnically diverse high school in California. The 85 students, who were predominantly Latino, were randomly assigned by computer to either the experimental or control condition. The experimental condition received the Think First training from a trained staff member on a twice-per-week basis over 4 weeks, whereas the control group received no anger management training. Among those students receiving the Think First training, the outcome data yielded a significant increase in academic achievement in an identified subject area and a significant decline in the number of detentions, office referrals, and suspensions.

Massey, Armstrong, and Boroughs (2003) studied the outcomes of the Think First program implemented in both class-based and pullout conditions. Class-based groups were made up of ninth-grade students enrolled in a peer mediation course and comprised 55% male and 45% female students. Sixty-four percent of the student participants were white non-Hispanic, and approximately 32% were in a free or reduced-cost lunch program. A nearly equivalent group made up students in the pullout condition. Teachers nominated students for the pullout program based on their history of disruptive and aggressive behaviors. Following the intervention, these researchers found significant improvements in both pullout and class-based groups in teacher ratings on a standardized rating scale of social, emotional, and behavioral functioning of the students and on a self-report measure of behavioral self-control for students in the pullout group. No significant improvements were found in parent ratings of student behavior, nor were changes found in disciplinary referrals.

The Think First program, although promising, is in need of continuing research and refinement. It is hoped that the manualized procedures contained in the following chapters will serve as stimuli for future research and publication so that the problems of this most needy population of students can be addressed most effectively.

CHAPTER 6

◆ ◆ ◆

Introduction to the Treatment Manual

◆

This chapter is followed by the complete procedures for implementing the revised Think First program. The curriculum is organized by *modules* that contain related content. *It is important that trainers not view the modules as a lock-step progression.* Each module will consist of multiple *meetings*. There is nothing to be gained by forging ahead to the next Module in order to follow an arbitrary or calendar timeline. Think First is not a class; it is a set of skills-training procedures that progress, linger, or recur, depending on the needs of the students involved. A figure range that indicates the approximate number of meetings for each module is provided on the first page of the module. *This range should be considered advisory only.* Shortened meetings, absenteeism, and, more important, the decision to extend training on a particular skill element, all contribute to how long the training group will last. It is suggested that trainers begin the intervention in the fall semester, allow for a minimum number of once-weekly meetings for the entire semester, and use the remainder of the year for follow-up booster sessions and progress monitoring. More frequent meetings (e.g., twice weekly) are at the discretion of the trainers, but they should be predicated on the needs of the students and not the school calendar. Anger and aggression management with adolescents is, in the vernacular, a "tough nut," and it deserves the requisite respect afforded by adequate time for the task.

Each module is organized in the following manner:

1. *Preparation.* This section contains information that the trainers need to consider prior to the meeting, such as needed supplies or useful reminders.

2. *Outcomes.* Each module has desirable learning outcomes that may be used to guide decisions about movement through the training elements. The *Outcomes* are

subdivided into *Knowledge Level* and *Skills Level*. Knowledge-level outcomes are those that are at the understanding or awareness level and are prerequisite for the more complex behavioral, skill-based outcomes. For example, understanding that anger has physiological, cognitive, and behavioral aspects is a knowledge-level outcome. However, the ability to use that knowledge in the implementation of a useful anger management strategy in the context of the general school setting is a *skill*. Consequently, an assessment of training outcomes must evaluate not only what students know, but what they are able to do. These outcomes should be viewed as guidelines only, with decisions to emphasize or de-emphasize one in favor of another for individual group members left to the trainers.

3. *Functional Vocabulary*. At the beginning of each module, terms and expressions are listed that are relevant to the training outcomes. Trainers are urged to teach the meaning and usages of these words and to model and encourage their use freely in the training. In any cognitive-behavioral intervention, it is critical to provide clients with vocabulary that not only helps them understand the constructs but also becomes available for their own use in their cognitive formulation of events. For instance, having the word "irritated" in one's vocabulary allows for the potential to label anger arousal at a more manageable intensity than if anger were construed only as a unitary, rage-level feeling.

4. *Comment*. This section contains introductory observations about the content of the module to come, as well as and necessary review of research relevant to the training procedures.

5. *Trainers' Hints*. Over the past decade trainers around the country, interns under my supervision, and I have acquired a wealth of insights and suggestions to help make Think First move more smoothly. *Trainers' Hints* is the section that contains "wheels that have already been invented" and is designed to provide first-time trainers with ideas and proactive strategies to assist in effectiveness and efficiency.

6. *Module Procedure*. This section contains the actual training procedures that are designed to lead to the expressed knowledge and skills outcomes. Much of the content from the original Think First (Larson & McBride, 1992) intervention that was the subject of the research discussed in Chapter 5 has been retained in this revision. Considerable expansion of those procedures has been made, and new training skills informed by subsequent research with aggressive youths have been added.

7. *Comprehension Checks at Decision Points*. A various intervals in the module, comprehension checks are inserted to assist trainers as they make decisions regarding when to progress to the next elements of training.

MEETING 1: COLLABORATIVE MENTORSHIP

The initial meeting is the first opportunity to begin the development of a rapport with the students that varies from what some may understand as the traditional helper–student relationship. When working with high-risk, externalizing adolescents in a skills-training modality, it is important that the trainers establish and cultivate a balanced relationship that is hierarchical but not authoritarian. The comparative social status of the adult leaders is undeniably superior, suitable to their age, position, and professional expertise, and this status should be kept overtly clear. Individual physical strength issues aside, the adult leaders hold significantly more power than the students do, and in the context of the group room the trainers are the adults in charge. Behavior on the part of any student that is disrespectful of this hierarchy, for example, inappropriate remarks or direct noncompliance, should be addressed immediately. However, the imbalance of power needs to be moderated if a fruitful relationship is to be developed.

I prefer to conceptualize the trainer–student relationship as more akin to that of a coach and pupil rather than that of the traditional therapist and client. Consider a golf professional who engages in a training relationship with an individual who wants to improve his or her game. The pupil arrives with an existing set of skills, and the coach listens to the training needs he or she expresses. For instance, the individual may say, "I've come to you because I want to fix my slice. It's ruining my game."

The professional will then assess the existing skills of the pupil and, using that information, proceed to help the pupil make the changes that will address the presenting problem:

"When is the slice most evident?"
"Are there some conditions in which it disappears?"
"What have you tried to correct it?"

Upon assessing the skills of the pupil, the professional may conclude that the slicing golf ball is only a symptom in a host of more systemic mistakes that lead up to it. However, the good golf professional always frames the golf lesson in terms of the pupil's concerns ("Let's work on that slice") and then skillfully uses his or her knowledge of setup and swing mechanics to allow the lesson to generalize to other aspects of the game. In this sense the teacher incorporates the training desires of the student and enters into collaboration with him or her to improve the golf game.

In a similar fashion, adolescent students arrive for anger and aggression management skills training with an existing repertoire of coping skills and, almost always, an explanation for their difficulties in the school building—for example, "The teachers never listen to my side." The effective skills trainer, like the effective golf professional, will incorporate and not dismiss this concern:

"When does this seem to occur most?"
"Are there times when the teachers do listen to you?"
"What have you tried to fix this problem?"

The skilled trainer attends to the student's conceptualization of the problem and holds in abeyance hypotheses about "what the real problem is." In this manner the trainer begins to cultivate a mutually respectful collaboration within the context of an imbalance of power. I refer to this balance between adult authority and student need as *collaborative mentorship*. Similar to the classic concept of "collaborative empiricism" (e.g., Beck, Rush, Shaw, & Emery, 1979) or "therapeutic alliance" (e.g., Meichenbaum, 2001) discussed in the adult cognitive-behavior literature, the trainer and student enter a reciprocal association that requires listening, understanding, and flexibility from both parties. In a group skills-training context, the trainers convey the message that each student's conceptualization of the problem is both affirmed and valued through regular directed inquiry and authentic role-play opportunities:

> "How did your concern that the teachers don't listen to your side of the story affect what happened this past week? Were there any incidents that you would like to share?"

Collaborative mentorship does not mean that the student "runs the show." My experience is that the typical adolescent with reactive–aggressive behaviors has a very narrow and egocentric problem conceptualization and, indeed, one that is quite prone to dramatic change in short periods of time. Whereas last week the student's explanation of the problem may have resided in teacher (mis)behavior, this week the finger is pointing at someone or something else. Competent trainers anticipate and subsume this rather predictable adolescent trait and use it to training advantage:

> "How can we use what we learned last week about considering consequences to help you with the problem you are now having with the gang kids near your locker?"

The knowledge and skills articulated in each module's training outcomes remain a constant, but the vehicle and context for their assimilation into the behavior of the students is fluid and linked to authentic concerns.

Rather than pointing out or becoming frustrated with the students' inconsistencies and flip-flops, an essential aspect of this manner of training is to assist them to see the possible relationships between their various problem conceptualizations. The trainers may conclude that a common element in a particular student's difficulties is impulsive behavior and seek to have the student recognize that commonality:

> "I was wondering if the problem that you were having with the teachers and the problem you are now having with the gang kids are the same in any way?"

Trainers who stick doggedly to their own agendas and ignore the student's conceptualization and experience of the problem increase the risk for low treatment involvement. In such circumstances the student may come to view the training as just another adult demand for behavioral change—often a lifelong bane—and respond with the resistance and noncompliance that has characterized previous intervention attempts from parents, teachers, and others.

CHALLENGE TASKS

At the close of every meeting, trainers should collaborate with individual students on a behavioral assignment to be met in the upcoming week. Most often the particulars of this "challenge task" will arise naturally out of the interactions in the meeting. For instance, a student may have described a problem with a teacher, confirmed a number of office referrals for misconduct at lunch, or admitted that the lost textbook for English has yet to be replaced. Trainers should assess the potential of the student to approach his or her problem and come to an agreement regarding what the student will do.

• Effort should be made to avoid having the student perceive this as just another "assignment" to evade with the usual litany of excuses. Rather than prescribe the task (e.g., "Why don't you . . . ?"or "Here's what I'd like you to do . . . "), attempt to elicit the behavior from the student less directly:

"Is there something you could do this week that might help?"
"I am wondering if you might have an idea about this?"
"Pretty tough situation. Is there anything you could do?"

• If the student fails to identify a behavior, trainers can become more direct:

"I was wondering if maybe you could. . . . "
"What might happen if you . . . ?"

• Avoid the use of the word "try" in the challenge task, as in "Okay, I'll try to be in all my classes." Indicate to the students that the task is something that the student can and will do. If necessary, reduce the difficulty, for example, "I will be in biology every day next week."
• When appropriate, challenge the student.

"I'm not certain you're ready for that yet."
"That sounds pretty hard. Should we think of something else?"

• Have fun. Wager points or candy bars against the successful task completion:

"I've got 5 points against your 1 that you can avoid an office referral next week!"

Trainers should maintain a notebook log of the challenge tasks for reference at the next meeting. A failed challenge task can be recycled in total, adjusted for difficulty, or held in abeyance for a later date.

MEETING STRUCTURE

Trainers will find that having a predictable structure for each meeting will be well received by the group members. The following structure has proved effective:

1. Greet students and verbally reinforce attendance.
2. Assign points for attendance and any completed hassle logs or other homework.
3. Allow members to fill out a hassle log on an event that occurred since the previous meeting.
4. Through active role play, address one or more of the most salient hassle-log issues, practicing new knowledge and skills, and award points for role-play participation.
5. Review knowledge and skills from previous meetings.
6. Introduce new training.
7. Assign challenge tasks.
8. Close with snack reinforcer and relaxation exercise.

ACKNOWLEDGMENT

Once again, I want to acknowledge the enormous influence that the work of Eva Feindler and her colleagues (Feindler & Ecton, 1986; Feindler et al., 1984, 1986) had on the intervention procedures contained in this Think First manual. Many of the training concepts and much of the structure and terminology of the first iteration of Think First were drawn from Feindler et al.'s groundbreaking group anger control work with adolescents. This revised manual retains a substantial portion of the original content, and, accordingly, my debt and gratitude continue.

VIDEOTAPE

A recently completed video that uses young actors to demonstrate many of the training concepts in Think First is available by contacting the author (*larsonj@uww.edu*).

THINK FIRST MEETING STRUCTURE

1. Greet students and verbally reinforce attendance.

2. Assign points for attendance and any completed hassle logs or other homework.

3. Allow members to fill out a hassle log on an event that occurred since the previous meeting.

4. Through active role play, address one or more of the most salient hassle-log issues, practicing new knowledge and skills, and award points for role-play participation.

5. Review knowledge and skills from previous meetings.

6. Introduce new training.

7. Assign homework or challenge tasks.

8. Close with snack reinforcer and relaxation exercise.

THINK FIRST TREATMENT INTEGRITY CHECKLIST

On a weekly basis, did the trainers:

☐ Provide points and verbal reinforcement for desirable behavior?

☐ Use the functional vocabulary and encourage its use by the students?

☐ Engage the students in practice of the training elements such that they were actively rehearsing the skills at least as much as they were discussing and listening?

☐ Collaborate on challenge tasks that were linked to authentic problem behaviors in school?

☐ Monitor progress with teacher/administrator/student feedback and use the data to make adjustments as called for?

MODULE I

♦ ♦ ♦

Introduction, Choices, and Consequences

♦

Approximate number of meetings: Four to five

PREPARATION

Chalkboard or whiteboard
Handout I.1 and Academic Self-Monitoring Form (Appendix I)
Spiral notebook for challenge task log
Poster board for writing behavioral rules
Point system designed and ready for explanation
Procedures for transition to and from the group in place
Snack available

OUTCOMES

Knowledge Level

1. Students will understand the purpose of the group and the reasons for their inclusion.
2. Students will understand the procedures and times for future meetings.
3. Students will understand the behavioral rules of the group and applicable point system.

4. Students will understand that most of the behaviors that they engage in are choice behaviors.
5. Students will understand the relationship between antecedent, behavior, and consequence.
6. Students will be able to articulate at least one prosocial reason for learning how to improve their own capacity for self-control in challenging situations.

Skill Level

1. Students will demonstrate successful group attendance and transition skills.
2. Students will identify and complete a challenge task.

FUNCTIONAL VOCABULARY

Confidentiality
Choice
Consequence

COMMENT

This is the introductory module; thus it is critical to get the students involved and invested right at the start. A welcoming and upbeat tone that communicates positive regard for each individual's decision to attend is important. In many circumstances, this hour may contain the most positive adult interactions the youth will have in the entire day. That said, it is equally important to have an established structure of behavioral expectations and to communicate it immediately. Some trainers are comfortable with a somewhat relaxed atmosphere, whereas others prefer a tighter structure. To a great extent, this is a function of the needs of the particular group of students being served. The youths have been referred due to problems with self-control; consequently, environmental assistance from the structure is often necessary and appreciated by all. Some groups clearly need more than others. When in doubt, start out tight, and loosen up as ongoing circumstances dictate.

The learning outcomes in this modules focus on helping the students begin to acquire a sense of control over and responsibility for personal behavior. The hostile attributional style of many reactive–aggressive youths—the tendency to overperceive the actions of others as hostile—inclines them to habitually place the responsibility for their own behavior on others. These students' locus of control (Rotter, 1966) tends to be highly external with regard to negative events that occur in their lives. My colleague and fellow trainer, Dennis Weerts, used to characterize them as "kids who wake up each day and act as if they are buffeted about by the winds of fate, out of control, just waiting for the next blast to push them into more trouble."

The issue of confidentiality is discussed in this module. Trainers are urged to familiarize themselves with relevant state and local statutes and policies, including issues such as mandated reporter obligations and duty to warn and protect.

TRAINERS' HINTS

Trainers' Hint I.1

It is quite common for group members to challenge the legitimacy of their presence in the group, and it is beneficial for trainers to address these issues early on. This discussion can be the first of potentially many that helps the youth learn to make choices based on obtaining desirable longer term outcomes rather than based on impulse fueled by temporary discomfort. Don't argue or threaten; simply state the facts. Following are some common challenges and suggested responses.

"I don't need this group."

1. "I believe that it is too early to make a decision like that. Right now, perhaps you'd rather not be here, but most of us are wary of new things. If you still feel the same way after a few meetings, we'll talk."

2. "You are right: You don't *need* it like you need air or water. You would still go on living if you were not in this group. The question to honestly ask yourself, however, is: Might what I learn in here be in my best interest? Emotionally healthy people generally do what they think to be in their best interests."

3. "I will agree with you when you can present me with report card and office disciplinary records that support that position. What I have indicates that you are moving away from—not toward—your stated goal."

"I'm not coming back next time."

1. "That choice is, of course, up to you. I will never drag you in here against your will. Every time you attend, you attend by choice. There are consequences for attending and consequences for not attending. I urge you to make the choice that brings you the consequences that you want. If you are unsure what they are, let's talk after group."

"You can't make me attend this group."

1. "Absolutely true. Nor can anyone else. Attending or not attending is entirely up to you. In addition, once you are here, staying or leaving is also up to you. One of the skills we will be working on in here is learning to predict consequences in order to make choices that work for you, not against you."

Trainers' Hint I.2

Model Rules for Think First Group

1. No physical contact between group members.
2. Allow everyone to express his or her opinion without interrupting.
3. What is said in here stays in here, except as explained by [trainer].
4. No racial or sexual slurs.
5. No group member put-downs, except in role plays.
6. Attend all meetings or have a valid excuse signed by an adult.

Trainers' Hint I.3

1. Consider bringing an array of snacks (three or four kinds of candy bars, single-serving bags of salty snacks, etc.) and have the group members decide on which two items will be available at the conclusion of each meeting and how much they will "cost" in points. Try to obtain the snacks through a community service grant from the local supermarket.
2. Obtain an in-school grant from the principal to purchase bookstore supplies and collaborate with the group members on their point value, or have them available noncontingently on an "as needed" basis.
3. Collect donations—gift certificates, free movie passes, and so forth—from local merchants and collaborate with the group members on their point value.
4. Arrange with the school kitchen staff for "extra dessert" or "extra pizza slice" certificates. Be certain they are counterfeit-proof and nontransferable!
5. Arrange with the principal for a "detention time reduction" certificate that the youth may use one time to get out of a school detention early. (Not all principals will go for this, and you need to be careful of alienating detention room staff. Consult ahead of time.)
6. Plan a group activity, such as a video movie and pizza day, lunch at a fast-food restaurant, or a visit to a local attraction, and assign a whole-group cumulative point requirement. This should be separate from individual reinforcers and should reflect the gross cumulative total, including those points expended on individual items during the course of the semester.

Trainers' Hint I.4

Institute a strict attendance and tardy policy. Brainstorm a point penalty for unexcused absence or repeated tardiness. Define what will constitute an excused absence (e.g., copy of official school absence slip or some other verifiable procedure.) Allow the student who is legitimately absent to be granted a minimum point allowance for that day (e.g., 2–3 points) so as not to fall too far behind.

Trainers' Hint I.5

Although the principal focus of Think First is on interpersonal behavior, the Academic Self-Monitoring form helps to remind everyone that the skills are being trained in the context of an academic environment in which one of the goals is to progress to the next grade. Self-monitoring programs work most effectively with students who are already motivated to make changes or to enact the desired behavior. Consequently, trainers should anticipate that some students, at least initially, will simply blow it off or "fake good" or "fake bad" merely to demonstrate that they are uncomfortable or unready to make the changes. Give them time. Generally avoid challenging the students' truthfulness; rather, simply give the form a brief review and make a comment of support or encouragement. Improving or maintaining positive interpersonal relationships with teachers is an important issue for students with problem behaviors. Advise students that the "positive comment to teacher" need only be a simple "Hi" or "Wassup, Mr. Jones" or any other friendly, student-initiated comment.

Trainers' Hint I.6

No meeting closing procedures are built into the text of this and the following modules. The reason is that meeting times vary and groups move at different rates. All modules require multiple meetings before the trainers believe that the group is ready to move on to the next module. Liberal use of informal and embedded comprehension checks on knowledge-level material as the group progresses will assist pacing decisions (e.g., "Robert, what did we say was meant by . . . ?"). Always begin each new meeting with a review and comprehension check from the previous meeting. Additionally, when in doubt, err on the side of additional time for continuing practice of skill-level content. (In real estate, the three most important words are: "Location. Location. Location." In skills training, the three most important words are: "Practice. Practice. Practice.") Before dismissing the group from any meeting, leave time for a snack and for reminders about any out-of-group generalization expectations (e.g., challenge tasks), set the next meeting time, and record earned points. After the first meeting only, provide an opportunity for a postgroup conference for any students who believe that they do not want to participate further in the group.

MODULE I PROCEDURE

Introduction

1. If they are unfamiliar with one another, have group members introduce themselves. Be certain that the trainers are aware of the youth's preferred name (e.g., "J. C." not "John"). Ask if necessary. It communicates respect.

2. Trainers should introduce themselves, including relevant professional history and why they have chosen to run this group. Make an effort to dispel any group members' belief that this is "just your job" and that is the only reason that you are with them today. It is likely that some have sat through the efforts of bored or burned-out counselors or probation officers before and have realistically low expectations. Communicate enthusiasm and a genuine outlook for positive change.

3. Remind group members of the purpose of this group:

"The purpose of this group is to help you achieve your personal achievement goals here in school. When we spoke individually, each of you told me that it was your long-term goal to graduate from high school (or pass the seventh/ eighth grade). We are here today because that goal might not be reached unless you learn some new skills to help you along. Our purpose here is to move you forward toward your personal goal." (See Trainers' Hint I.1.)

Discuss "Housekeeping" Issues

1. Meeting times and places
2. Transition to and from group (e.g., hall passes, late slips)
3. How any missed class work will be made up
4. Absentee or tardy policy (see Trainers' Hint I.4)

Brainstorm a Set of Behavioral Rules with the Group (see Trainers' Hint I.2)

The rules should be few in number and cover the most likely contingencies. It is important that the group members are fully engaged in the process so that there is a sense of ownership. Once they are decided on, the trainers should write the rules on a poster board. The following prompts are useful:

1. What about physical contact?
2. What about put-downs?
3. What about language?
4. What about confidentiality?
5. What about "signing" (if there are gang issues)?
6. What about attendance?

Explain the Point System

A functional point system must have value to the group members. They must see the "point" as a *secondary reinforcer*; that is, exchangeable at a later time for a desired commodity or activity. If the individuals do not value the commodity or activity, the system will have no effect, and it may even contribute negatively (See Trainers' Hint I.3). Points may be earned through such behaviors as:

1. On-time attendance
2. Completion of hassle-log or successful challenge task
3. Role-play participation

The following are trainer-judgment point awards:

4. Cooperative peer interaction (assisting, supporting, empathizing)
5. A spontaneous or responsive insight that indicates the youth was attentive and reflecting seriously on the issue at hand
6. Improvement in group conduct from initial baseline level
7. Exhibition of self-control following peer provocation

As an option, trainers may choose to link group points to positive general school behavior. For example, points may be awarded for (1) a week without an office referral, (2) an improved report card, (3) a high grade on a test or paper, or (4) any other positive academic or social behavior considered worthy.

Discuss Issues of Confidentiality

Trainers should be familiar with applicable legal and ethical code guidelines and obligations, including mandated reporter requirements. The meaning and limitations of "confidentiality" should be thoroughly discussed. Under what circumstances will the trainers reveal to others what was said in the group? Explain the rationale for the expectation that what is said in the group should not be repeated by group members to others outside of the group. Why do we have this rule? What would happen if we did not have this rule? Ask if maintaining confidentiality will be difficult for any of the members and brainstorm possible solutions if necessary. Recommend that group members who have personal concerns unrelated to the training share them first with the trainers in private.

Discuss Individual Collaborative Training Goals

Trainers should take this opportunity to initiate the training collaboration with the group members. This is asking the students to admit to a certain vulnerability, so trainers should be aware that some may not be ready. This element may be repeated in later meetings as necessary. Introduce it in a manner such as this:

> "This is a group about helping you to meet your goals in school. We have many ideas about how to help you, but they are useless unless we know what you want to accomplish. We know that all of you want to graduate [or pass to the next grade], but what do you see as the biggest problem in the way of that goal? If you could make that problem magically disappear today, how would you do it? Students from other groups that we have worked with have identified problems such as:
>
> > My temper gets me into too many hassles.
> > The teachers never listen to my side of the story.
> > Other kids get me into trouble.
> > The principal has it in for me.
>
> "We would like to take this opportunity to have you think about a problem or problems that you would like help on in this group. Take a couple of minutes now to think about it, and then we will go around the group."

Allow time for reflection, then move from student to student and write down their expressed problems on a pad of paper. Clarify and behavioralize the problems with:

> "Do I hear you saying that . . . ?"
> "My understanding is that you believe that. . . . "
> "Help me to understand better. Is it that . . . ?"

Trainers should avoid adding their own opinions or suggesting other problems at this time. However, if the student is unable to articulate a problem but is clearly attempting, then adult assistance is appropriate. Some students may deny that they have any problems in school and that it is other individuals in the building who must change. Trainers should phrase such problems in terms of the student's obligation to function in the face of others' fallibility:

> "Do I hear you saying that your biggest problem is trying to stay out of trouble in classrooms where the teachers don't control the students?"

Some students may deny the existence of any problems in school whatsoever, even in the face of overwhelming data to the contrary. Trainers should use the preceding clarifying questions to try to elicit something. However, the first meeting is not the time for confrontation on this issue. Trainers are advised to reinforce the student for reflecting on the subject with verbal praise and move to the next student.

Trainers should commit these expressed problems to memory and regularly refer to them in the course of the training. In time, it may become clear to both trainer and student that the initially expressed problem is not the most salient or that it is only one problem among many. In such cases, trainers should simply reframe the collaboration in terms of addressing the new concerns.

Academic Self-Monitoring

Trainers should distribute copies of the Academic Self-Monitoring form and explain its use to the students. This form is designed to help the students pay attention to classroom behaviors that contribute positively to academic achievement. Attendance, homework return, active participation by asking questions, and positive relationships with teachers are all subject to self-monitoring. Distribute this form at the onset of every meeting. It should require no more than about 3–5 minutes' time (see Trainers' Hint I.5).

Teach "Personal Choice Behavior"

Many adolescents with problem behavior think of "choice" as the process of selecting between two or more personally desirable activities or commodities. For example, "Shall I go to the mall or watch a video? Order curly fries or regular fries? Buy a red shirt, a black one, or both?" *Undesirable* choice behavior is typically categorized under "have to" or "forced to." For example, "I have to go to school" or "My parents force me to be in before eleven on school nights." In both of these instances, the choice is still there. The youth could choose not to attend school or choose to stay out past 11. The variable is the aversive consequence that may ensue. This leads the youth to think, erroneously, that there really is not a choice. In this exercise, the objective is to provide the group members with the insight that almost all day-to-day behavior is *personal choice behavior* (PCB)—even behavior that has the sole purpose of avoiding a negative consequence.

1. Ask for lists of behaviors that the group members freely choose to do on a daily basis and write them on the chalkboard. It will likely contain enjoyable, personally preferred behaviors such as chatting on the computer, hanging out with friends, eating good food, and the like.

2. Ask for a second list of behaviors that they do on a daily basis that they do *not* do by choice, and write these on the chalkboard. This list may contain such behaviors as going to school and doing chores.

3. Challenge their belief that they are forced to engage in any nonchoice behavior by asking them to convince you that doing chores, coming to school, doing homework, and so forth is really not personal choice behavior. Ask: Is it possible for you to not do it? Do you ever not do it? If so, it is a personal choice behavior.

4. Emphasize that if you are locked in a room or a cell you have to choose to stay, but that most daily behavior that is not controlled by physical means is personal choice behavior. Discuss some examples of personal choice behaviors:

   a. Attending school or skipping school
   b. Doing homework or not doing homework
   c. Complying with a teacher request or not complying with a teacher request
   d. Initiating an assault or not initiating an assault
   e. Seeking revenge or not seeking revenge

Discuss Consequences

1. Ask: What do all PCBs have in common? (They each produce a consequence.) Explain that a *consequence* is what happens after a personal choice behavior and that consequence can be positive or negative for the person.

2. Consequences can be short term or long term: For the list of PCBs discussed earlier, ask the group to come up with short-term and long-term consequences for each. For example, the short-term positive consequences of skipping school include having fun with friends and avoiding boring classes. Are there any long-term positive consequences? What are the short-term negative consequences for choosing to attend school? What are the long-term positive consequences? Are there any long-term negative consequences? Pursue this line of questioning for the following behaviors:

   a. Attending school or skipping school
   b. Doing homework or not doing homework
   c. Complying with a teacher request or not complying with a teacher request
   d. Initiating an assault or not initiating an assault
   e. Seeking revenge or not seeking revenge

COMPREHENSION CHECK DECISION POINT

(Proceed in module or return for additional work.)

   1. Confidentiality
   2. Personal choice behavior
   3. Consequences

The A–B–C Method (see Handout I.1)

Explain how any angry conflict situation can be looked at or analyzed in terms of:

- A—What triggered the problem? (What led up to it?)
- B—What did you do? (What was your response to "A"?)
- C—What were the consequences for everyone?

Trainers should provide examples from their own lives, citing both good and bad consequences. Examples such as anger while driving a car that led to a traffic ticket will help to bring the construct to a concrete level. Use abundant visual aids. Choreographed examples with a co-trainer are effective. For example:

- A—*Something happens*: "I was on my way to work one day and got stuck behind a very slow-moving driver."
- B—*What I choose to do*: "I leaned on the horn and flashed my lights. When he finally turned off, I was so angry at him, I sped off so quickly that I forgot about the speed limit."
- C—*What are the consequences?*: "I got pulled over for speeding two blocks from school."

The trainers should now solicit anger incidents from the students. The trainers should first model the format of reporting. Each component should be preceded with its introduction. For example:

- A—*Something happens*: "I let Robert look at my new watch in the locker room after gym and he dropped it on the floor."
- B—*What I choose to do*: "I shoved him against the locker and called him a name."
- C—*What are the consequences*: "He tried to hit me back and we got in a fight and both got suspended."

Encourage students to recall an angry incident *in the school*. Remind those students who give examples that glorify their aggressive anger that you appreciate their honesty and are glad that they now have the opportunity to learn greater self-control. It will be hard to avoid the discussion becoming one of "who is more aggressive than whom." Note with emphasis the negative consequences ("C") of aggression. Group members will often try to outdo their peers, and there are liable to be a lot of "high fives" going around and precious little concern for consequences, or the consequence will be glossed over or even lied about. This is to be expected in some groups, as there is still considerable concern for peer status. *One of the goals as trainer is to slowly move self-control, or "keeping your cool," into a "status" position. Patience is required.* In fight situations, emphasize that the student "chose to fight" rather than was "forced to fight," even though you may acknowledge that when you were 15, you might have made the same choice.

COMPREHENSION CHECK DECISION POINT

(Proceed to next module or return for additional work.)

1. Can each student describe, with understanding, the A–B–C sequence and provide an example?
2. Can each student provide at least one prosocial reason for learning how to improve their own capacity for self-control in challenging situations?

MODULE II

♦ ♦ ♦

Hassle Log and Anger Reducers

♦

Approximate number of meetings: Three to four

PREPARATION

Hassle logs copied for handout (Handout II.2)
Pencils
Poster paper and marker or chalkboard
Multidimensional School Anger Inventory (Appendix F)
Snack available

OUTCOMES

Knowledge Level

1. Students will know how to complete a hassle log self-monitoring procedure.
2. Students will be able to provide a definition of anger.
3. Students will understand that an individual's anger level can be described on a continuum of intensity, from mild to very strong.
4. Students will understand that anger has a physiological aspect that can be self-perceived, monitored, and controlled.
5. Students will be able to describe their own physiological responses to increased anger levels.

Skill Level

1. Students will be able to demonstrate one or more palliative anger reducers in the group setting.

FUNCTIONAL VOCABULARY

Irritated
Annoyed
Furious
Anger cue

COMMENT

It is useful for trainers to conceptualize anger as having cognitive, phenomenological, and behavioral components: what the students believe, how they feel physically, and what they do. Anger is, in part, the experience of an internal arousal mechanism that has perceivable physiological effects on an individual (Novaco, 1979; see also Feindler, 1995; Larson & Lochman, 2001). In this module, the students are introduced to this insight and trained to become aware of their own physiological experiences as cues or signals to initiate anger control strategies. In this way, students learn to exert more control over impulsive anger–aggression responses. The idea of anger cues is an occasionally difficult concept for them to grasp but an important one nonetheless. Anger arousal is a predominant precursor to many problematic forms of adolescent aggression. Consequently, it is important for students to have a phenomenological sense of what their own escalating anger "feels" like so that they can initiate anger control efforts. Trainers may find that some group members have problems labeling their own feeling states in general and may require additional work in affective education prior to concentrating on anger. For example, how does feeling anxious differ from feeling angry? How can you tell when you are feeling one and not the other? In terms of affect regulation, group members often have techniques for calming themselves when nervous or fearful, or even procedures for keeping tears at bay during times of sadness; however, most have considerably less skill recognizing and controlling anger.

In this module, group members are asked to express their own conceptualizations of what conditions or persons in the school seem to occasion their anger, and trainers should attend carefully to them. In particular, note should be made of those students who express highly elevated and emotion-laden demands that others not challenge their senses of puffed-up self-esteem (e.g., "If some dork disses me or looks at me funny, I want to kill them!"). In some highly aggressive individuals, this threat to their own elevated self-concept is often the trigger for anger and aggression (Bandmaster, Smart, & Boden, 1996).

TRAINERS' HINTS

Trainers' Hint II.1

Be certain to review previously trained material at the onset of each new meeting. Help the group members to understand the connections as you progress in the training. For instance, the recognition of anger cues happens during the "A—Something Happens" portion of the A–B–C construct discussed in Module I. A provocation or frustrating experience stimulates the arousal mechanism, and the decision to control the arousal and the behavior that accompanies it happens at the "B—What I Choose to Do" portion of the sequence. The students should have the insight that anger control is largely personal choice behavior.

Trainers' Hint II.2

The enclosed hassle log (Handout II.2) is a model adapted from Feindler and Ecton (1986), but it can and should be readapted to fit local circumstances, including school locales in which aggression is frequent. Ease of completion is the key; problematic adolescents are unlikely to expend a great deal of academic energy on such a task. It is recommended that a reinforcement point for each successfully completed hassle log be granted. Ideally, students leave with a blank hassle log after the group is over, fill it out shortly after a conflict event, and return with it for the next meeting. This procedure should be attempted following the meeting that introduces the hassle log. Experience has shown, however, that this expectation is generally unrealistic. It is a rare student who leaves with a hassle log in hand and returns with it completed at the next meeting. What happens most frequently is that the group members arrive, ask for new sheets, and fill them out before or during the review. This is not all bad, as it is an attempt at compliance and is best not discouraged. With self-contained groups, such as a classroom for students with emotional-behavioral disabilities, we made sure a stack was left with the teacher. Trainers may want to consider providing the administrator in charge of discipline with some hassle logs to retain in his or her office. Using the logs during a disciplinary encounter with a group member can serve as a generalization aid.

Trainers' Hint II.3

The hassle logs are stimuli for role plays, a chance to get the group members on their feet and practicing newly trained concepts. The student/author should play him- or herself, and other group members and trainers should play the "supporting roles." Some shyness and hesitancy are expected early on, but they need to get over it. Point reinforcers help. Trainers should press for realism as much as possible, as lazy, silly, or halfhearted role plays waste time. It is essential that the role plays *always* rehearse an adaptive, nonaggressive response to the provocation. Never give in to student pressure to role-play the original, maladaptive response.

Trainers' Hint II.4

Research indicates that highly aggressive youths tend to overlabel emotional arousal as anger (Lochman, White, & Wayland, 1991). In this module, the group members are asked to understand anger as existing on a continuum of intensity and are taught language to match those levels of intensity. The further goal is to train the students to become aware of the arousal cues and then to give them a functional cognitive label (e.g., "irritated") that may encourage a lower level, more manageable anger response. If "anger" is defined in a group member's mind only as a fury reaction, then the arousal cue is much more likely to lead him or her to that level. Trainers are encouraged to identify and teach a suitable vocabulary and to model and use that vocabulary throughout the training. For example, rather than observe that a group member became "angry," trainers might observe that the youth became "annoyed."

Trainers' Hint II.5

We have occasionally found the visual of an "anger thermometer" to be useful in helping youths to see anger expression on a continuum. Draw a simple thermometer on a chalkboard or on poster board, with the 212-degree mark at the top ("boiling rage!"), then moderate downward, using the new vocabulary, to 98.6 degrees ("calm, not even mildly annoyed"). Have the students identify on the thermometer where their anger would be following some incident.

Trainers' Hint II.6

Depending on the response, this might be a good time to discuss what we have come to call the "I just ignore them" cop-out. Students will express this particular technique to the trainer as if it were real. The reason is that because they have been told all their lives by concerned adults that it is real technique. From a practical standpoint, however, it is quite impossible to "ignore" an incoming sensory stimulation, assuming functional sensory systems. Point out that by "ignore," the student really means that he or she is choosing to attend to something else. They are probably self-instructing or self-distracting (active) rather than ignoring (passive). Probe with the students just what they are *doing* to "ignore," and reinforce their skill.

Trainers' Hint II.7

Our experience with boys in particular is that they will struggle with the whole notion of recognizing and using anger cues. Girls are typically socialized to be more attendant to their own emotional situations and can generally describe their physiological reactions with greater insight. This module is designed only to introduce them to the concept of anger cues, not to train them in using cues effectively. That will come over time in the intervention. Once trainers believe that the students have acquired the concept at a knowledge level, then it is time to move on.

Trainers' Hint II.8

Some trainers have built in a deep-breathing relaxation period at the end of each meeting, with remarkable acceptance from the students. Try it!

MODULE II PROCEDURE

Introduce the Hassle Log (Handout II.1)

At this point, the trainers introduce the self-monitoring procedure, called the "hassle log." This device has a number of purposes:

1. It serves as a monitoring device that will record how conflicts are handled during the week.
2. It serves as a memory aid to assist students in their recollection and organization of conflict during the week.
3. It is used as a basis for role play in the group.

Trainers should go over the hassle log, section by section, and then have the group members fill out their own for a recent conflict event. Ask volunteers to present their hassle logs, and answer any remaining procedural questions (see Trainers' Hints II.2 and II.3). It is productive to have a hassle log review near the beginning of each meeting, as it can serve as a stimulus for training that involves authentic group members' issues.

Understanding Anger

Trainers should conduct a discussion on the meaning of "anger." On the chalkboard, write "anger."

1. Trainers should model first, and then ask group members to recall the last time that they were really angry at something. Stress *feeling* really angry rather than showing aggression.

"Think of a time when you felt really, really angry. What was happening?"

2. Trainers should attempt to elicit an insight into commonalities:

"What is one thing that all of our anger incidents have in common with one another?"

The answer will frequently be that a student's anger arose because someone said or did something that they did not want them to. *Anger is often a reaction to the student's unreasonable demand that other people should always behave as he or she wants them to behave.* For example, we don't want others to call us names, and so when they do, we become angry at them. We don't want others to deny us privileges, treat us unfairly, or physically assault us, and so when they do, we become angry at them.

3. Trainers should seek agreement on what the purpose or function of anger is:

"If the purpose of the feeling of fear is to protect us from harm, what's the purpose of the feeling of anger? Why do people to get angry?"

Responses may include: to scare other people and stop them from messing with you; to get what you want; to send a message; to make people, such as your children, behave. Ask:

"When is anger *good* anger, and when is anger *bad* anger?"

Examples:

> *Good*: When you get angry at a personal or societal wrong and work to change it nonviolently (e.g., Martin Luther King, Rosa Parks, Cesar Chavez and Dolores Huerta, Bobby Kennedy, Betty Friedan). Stress that controlled anger can be a very useful feeling as a stimulus to act for positive change in life. Controlled anger can also help you protect yourself: Martial arts and boxing champions don't lose their tempers in a match.
> *Bad*: When anger causes you to become aggressive or cruel and to hurt someone else even though you don't mean to.

4. Trainers should provide the insight that anger can be expressed on a continuum of intensity. *It is important to teach and use the vocabulary with regularity* (see Trainers' Hint II.4). Have the group come up with words that mean the same thing as anger, and place them on a continuum from least intense to most intense. Assist as necessary, and write the terms on a poster board or chalkboard. Examples:

Less: Irritated, annoyed, bothered, peeved, upset, bummed, pissed
More: Furious, enraged, livid, incensed

- Read selected items from the Multidimensional School Anger Inventory (Appendix F) and ask students to use the anger word that best describes their feeling following each provocation. (See Trainers' Hint II.5.)
- Model and ask for personal examples of events that have occasioned "irritation" and compare them with events that have occasioned "fury" or "rage."
- Compare the consequences following low-intensity and high-intensity anger incidents.

Anger Cues

Trainers should indicate that an important aspect of anger control is recognizing the hints or cues that the body sends that signal anger is on the rise.

1. The trainers should draw parallels to other feelings that students commonly encounter:

"What does your body feel like when you start to get nervous about something?"
"What does your body feel like when you start to become more and more embarrassed?"

2. Have students discuss what they do to calm themselves when they are afraid or nervous. (Note any use of self-instruction for later parallels.) Describe a scenario in which the student is at a basketball free-throw line with two shots and 1 second left on the clock. He or she needs to make the first free throw to tie and then another to win the game. The crowd is trying to make the player nervous. How does the player know that he or she is getting nervous? What does the player do to remain calm? How does the player keep the crowd from triggering his or her anxiety? (See Trainers' Hint II.6.)

3. Point out that anger cues are *warning signs in the body* that occur during the "A—Something Happens" aspect of the A–B–C sequence described earlier. They are signals from the body that it is time to control anger. (See Handout II.2.)

4. Using Handout II.2 as a visual aid, trainers should describe a personal scenario in which they recognized their anger cues and controlled their anger (e.g., consider the immediate anger arousal that often comes with being cut off on the highway, the physiological cues (flushing, accelerated heartbeat), and the decision to calm down rather than chase the culprit down the highway). Trainers should emphasize and describe their own anger cues.

5. Ask students to identify some of their own common anger cues. Some examples include muscle tension, blood rushing to face, heartbeat acceleration, and increased breathing rate.

> "How can you tell that you are becoming angrier? What does it feel like inside for you?"

It may be helpful to suggest that the students visualize and describe a recent situation in school in which they could feel themselves becoming increasingly angry.

6. Using Handout II.2 as a visual aid, trainers should have each student describe an actual A–B–C sequence of a provoking incident, the cues for anger, what the student did to control the anger, and the consequences.

7. Point out that getting in touch with the cues for or warning signs of anger is a critical step in getting the self-control necessary to avoid "losing your temper." It is important to get the students to begin thinking about anger and aggression as a sequential process (i.e., antecedents, behavior, consequences). (See Trainers' Hint II.7.)

Anger Reducers

Now that students are starting to become aware of their anger cues, they can begin to make use of anger reduction techniques to help them increase their self-control. Stress that the purpose of anger reducers is to *give the student time to decide how to respond most effectively.* Anger reducers calm the student down enough to allow time for considering an alternative. They help prevent the impulsive aggression. Students may feel uneasy and embarrassed when asked to rehearse the simple anger reducers given here. The trainer should be prepared for this and provide a clear model of the behavior desired.

1. Trainers should role-play a provoking incident *plus* anger cues *plus* anger reducer. For instance, ask a student to get up to sharpen his or her pencil and refuse to return to his or her seat when asked by the trainer. Trainers should then talk their way through the anger cues ("I can feel my heartbeat accelerate. I can feel the blood rushing to my face. I am thinking angry thoughts about that student"), then proceed to the anger reducer being modeled. Point out that the two anger reducers that will be introduced (following) can be accomplished privately, without anyone knowing about it.

2. Trainers should note that these anger reducers are for use in situations in which quick decision making is not critical but "best interest" decision making is. They are for use in situations in which the student can recognize the anger cues and do something to keep anger at the "irritated or annoyed" level, rather than becoming "furious."

Anger Reducer 1: Deep Breathing

Explain that taking slow, deep breaths can help in maintaining control in response to anger-provoking situations. The idea is to avoid the hyperoxygenating that comes with rapid breathing, a common anger cue. Point out that basketball players frequently use this technique at the foul line to calm themselves before attempting a shot. The technique is accomplished by:

1. A long, slow diaphragmatic inhalation through the nose (the abdomen should push out);
2. Immediate exhale, slowly.
3. During exhale, think the word "Reee-laa-xxx."
4. Continue to exhale slowly and repeat.

Trainers should assist the students in practicing this technique until each can accomplish it without outside assistance from the trainers. (See Trainers' Hint II.8.)

Anger Reducer 2: Backward Counting

Point out that this technique can be done silently or in a whisper. In some instances, it will help to turn away from whomever or whatever is provoking the student's anger. The student should start from 100 and move backward by 3's (e.g., 100, 97, 94, 91, 88, . . .). This sequence of odd numbers requires the mind to occupy itself more fully than simple rote backward counting.

3. Provide opportunities for the students to rehearse these techniques with one another. Use completed hassle logs when possible. Trainers will find that the students will be very creative in their role play. Keep them focused on realistic, school-related situations. It is critically important that the students believe in the merits of the techniques; they will not adopt new behaviors that they believe are silly or foolish for them. Trainers should also remember the importance of practice, practice, practice!

Some possible situations for student role-play are as follows:

- A teacher is being critical of your behavior, and he or she just keeps going on and on and on. . . .
- You are in class taking an important test, and you see another student mouth an obscenity at you.
- A teacher verbally blames you for something you didn't do and ignores you when you try to explain.
- Some kids are quietly teasing you about your new haircut in class to see if they can get you angry.

COMPREHENSION CHECK DECISION POINT

(Proceed to next module or return for additional work.)

1. Can each student provide a useful definition of anger?
2. Does each student understand anger as a continuum of feeling intensity?
3. Can each student articulate the need for recognition and use of anger cues?
4. Can each student demonstrate both trained anger reducers and identify a school situation in which either one would be useful?

MODULE III

♦ ♦ ♦

Anger Triggers
and Attribution Retraining

♦

Approximate number of meetings: Three to five

PREPARATION

Progress Monitoring Report forms copied
Handout III.1 copied for each student

OUTCOMES

Knowledge Level

1. Students will be able to identify their most problematic direct (external) anger provocations within the school setting.
2. Students will understand the meaning of the term "thought trigger" and be able to differentiate it from the term "anger trigger."
3. Students will be able to describe how a thought trigger can contribute to anger escalation.
4. Students will be able to describe a variety of potential thought triggers.
5. Students will understand how ascribing intent inaccurately can lead to anger and aggression.
6. Students will be able to describe facial features and body postures associated with anger or hostility.

Skill Level

1. Students will be able to demonstrate understanding of anger cues and anger reducers in the context of their own hassle-log incidents.
2. Students will show an ability to evaluate the intent of a potential provocation through the use of a "stop and think" technique paired with an anger reducer.

FUNCTIONAL VOCABULARY

Trigger
"Awfulizing"
Overgeneralization
Intention
Hostile

COMMENT

In the meetings for this module, the students will start to identify persons, events, and situations in the school setting that regularly and predictably occasion their anger and aggression ("anger triggers"). In the A–B–C sequence, this is still within the "A—Something Happens" element, and its relationship to the previous training in anger cue recognition is evident. Prior knowledge of high-risk situations allows the student the potential to exert some anticipatory control. For instance, a student may identify a certain lunchroom monitor or group of students as persons who appear to provoke his or her anger, and, armed with that insight, the student can actually engage in some form of preventive behavior. These meetings are also the first opportunity for the trainers to help students become aware of their own internal self-talk or belief statements and their possible contribution to anger ("thought triggers"). This is an essential insight, for it sets up the internal self-instruction techniques to follow. Some students will have a hard time being asked to "think about their thinking," and for a few younger students, delays in cognitive development may make it all the more difficult.

One of the crucial points associated with angry, reactive aggression has to do with what has been called "hostile attributional bias." From a practical standpoint, an attribution can be thought of as an individual's explanation for the occurrence of some event. Many chronically aggressive youths have a frequent tendency to misattribute a hostile intent where a benign one may have existed. In essence, they cognitively create anger triggers (e.g., "He did that on purpose!") from the same events that typically less aggressive youth would not (e.g., "He did it accidentally").

Although most of the literature in this area currently focuses on younger children, it clearly has applied value with adolescents. (For a discussion of this mechanism with adolescents, trainers should review Dodge et al., 1990, and the relevant section in Chapter 3 of this book.) These meetings provide the students with opportunities to examine the possibility of alternative attributional intent as a technique of anger and aggression control.

TRAINERS' HINTS

Trainers' Hint III.1

This is the time in the training to initiate the Progress Monitoring Report (see Appendix E). It is recommended that these forms be completed for each student in selected classes at least every other week *for the duration of the training*. Trainers should decide whether to have the group members take responsibility for the form distribution and return or to eliminate the student as middle person entirely and distribute directly to the teachers. The completed forms should be maintained by the trainers and, if possible, converted to graph form for student review.

Trainers' Hint III.2

As with each new meeting, trainers should begin this new module with a review of previous knowledge and skills and address evident weak areas. In hassle-log role plays, integrate knowledge of anger cues and anger reducers, whether or not the student actually used them during the actual event, and continue to frame anger or aggression encounters with the A–B–C sequence.

Trainers' Hint III.3

Anger triggers can be highly idiosyncratic and very culturally based. Students' experiences within their own cultural group incline them toward trigger sensitivities that may not be shared by members of different cultural groups. Trainers working in multicultural situations are urged to familiarize themselves with research pertaining to the students whom they serve. Useful reviews of this literature may be found in Matsumoto (2001a, 2001b).

When modeling anger triggers, trainers should use school-related issues. Frame the example in the A–B–C sequence. For instance: "When I was a ninth grader, there was a junior who used to make fun of my clothes by calling me 'country' in front of my friends. So, 'A,' I would be by my locker and I would see this kid coming. I could feel my face start to get hot and my anger rising just seeing him, even before he said anything. He was an anger trigger for me."

Trainers' Hint III.4

The thought-triggers exercises border somewhat on rational cognitive-restructuring principles, but trainers with expertise in rational–emotive behavior therapy (REBT) are advised to avoid disputation techniques and simply elicit the general insight. Once the term "thought trigger" enters the group's lexicon, then trainers are encouraged to regularly make reference to it as the group members discuss their conflict situations around the school. For example, as a youth is describing a sequence from his hassle log that led to an anger incident, the trainer should be asking, "What were your thought triggers when _____ happened?" The subsequent role play should include the alternative, non-anger-provoking thoughts.

Trainers' Hint III.5

Attribution retraining as a focus of anger and aggression management training is clearly in its infancy, and there is no compelling current research to support its efficacy with adolescents. It is included in this training manual because it has shown promise with younger populations and because it is a logical extension of the thought-trigger insights. Biased attributions in reactive–aggressive youths are often the precursors to impulsive retaliatory aggression. If the attribution of hostile intent goes unchallenged, the youth will proceed to deal with the interaction as if it were true (e.g., "He did mean to provoke me"). Training must first challenge the youth's firmly held belief in the infallibility of his or her appraisal capacity for the intentions of others and then attempt to train enough impulse control to allow for a less biased attribution to be considered. No easy task, this! It is recommended that at least two meetings be dedicated to this aspect of the training and that the insights be revisited when they are salient in future role plays.

Trainers' Hint III.6

Trainers can augment the skills training associated with reading facial expressions and body posture with photographs clipped from magazines. Trainers with knowledge of feature films on video may also choose to use relevant clips as training aids. An Internet search with the key words "facial expressions" and "body language" can also turn up some useful material that can be downloaded.

Trainers' Hint III.7

The insertion of the words "stop and think" serve as self-instruction designed to inhibit impulsive responding and should not be skipped over or denigrated in the training. They should initially be stated loudly and clearly. After a few role plays, the students may be allowed to mouth them silently.

MODULE III PROCEDURE

Anger Triggers

Remind students that each conflict situation has (A) something that triggers some-one's (B) angry behavior, leading to some kind of (C) consequence. Tell them that today we are going to list all the "triggers" we encounter in school on the chalk-board.

Write the words "ANGER TRIGGERS" on a chalkboard or poster board. Observe that anger triggers are people, places, or events that seem to spark angry feelings in some of us almost all of the time.

1. Anger triggers can be what some people do or say (e.g., the way a particular adult or student in the school talks to you or engages you with their nonverbal behaviors, such as eye-rolling or other signs of perceived disrespect). Anger triggers can also be general circumstances, such as a particularly difficult or frustrating class (see Trainer's Hint III.3).

2. Trainers should model examples from their own experience first (see Trainers' Hint III.3). They should note that this is a brainstorming session, so all should refrain from criticizing another's anger trigger. If at least one person is angered by some person or event, then it is a valid contribution. With adults in the school, ask, "What is it that _____ does that triggers your anger?" Stimulate responses with:

"What happens in school that triggers your anger?"
"Can teachers/administrators/hall aides trigger anger?"
"Is there anyone you know in school whose behavior triggers your anger almost every day?"
"Do you know people who seem to have more anger triggers than other people? Do you know some people who do not seem to have any?"

3. In the meeting, have the students complete new hassle logs on their most powerful anger trigger in the school and their most troublesome recent encounter with that trigger. In the role plays, have the students identify their anger cues and use either of the anger reducers (breathing or backward counting).

4. Have the students identify their own possible preventative behaviors that might be effective relative to that trigger. For example:

"How can you change your normal habits so as to avoid that person?"
"How can you use anger reducers before encountering him or her?"
"How can you use anger reducers during an encounter with him or her?"

Thought Triggers

1. Point out to the students that sometimes we can trigger our own anger by thinking anger-triggering thoughts to ourselves about what we believe someone says or does. These are called "thought triggers." Ask:

"Is seeing two other students talking together enough to trigger most students' anger?" (not normally).

"What might cause it to become an anger trigger?" (If you think they are talking negatively about you).

2. Provide students with a model from the trainers' own experience. A possible role play might be the following: The teacher has given a clear instruction that there will be no getting out of seats to sharpen pencils during the test. A student comes in late and misses that instruction. Later the student goes to the pencil sharpener. Trainers should model a "think aloud" procedure along the lines of:

"What's the matter with him?"
"I clearly stated no pencil sharpening!"
"He is trying to challenge my authority in here again!"
"These kids never listen!" etc.

Which was the anger trigger? The student or the teacher's beliefs about the student?

3. Help the students to identify common thought triggers that can increase anger during a frustrating or irritating situation and alternative thoughts to control anger. Trainers should distribute Handout III.1, "Common Thought Triggers," and repeat the following anger-provoking thought triggers aloud. Ask the group to discuss and provide more helpful alternatives. Remember to keep them related to issues in the school (adapted from Meichenbaum, 2001; see Trainers' Hint III.3).

- *"Awfulizing" triggers*: These are thought triggers that exaggerate the unpleasantness of situations and make them worse than they really are.
  "I can't stand the way he does that/says that!"
  Alternative: I don't like that, but I can handle it.
  "This is the worst thing that could ever happen!"
  Alternative: It's not the end of the world, but it's very frustrating.
- *Demanding triggers*: These are thought triggers that create "demands" out of wants or preferences, as if everyone ought to always do just what we demand that they do, and when they don't, we get angry.
  "He should not say that! He should not do that!"

Alternative: He can say and do what he wants. If I don't like it, I have choices.

Alternative: I don't know why he said/did that. Maybe I should ask him.

- *Overgeneralized triggers*: These are thought triggers that cause us to blow things way out of proportion and that are not really true. These triggers use such words as "always," "never," "everything," and "everybody" to describe what is really much more specific to a given situation.

  "He's always hassling me and never leaves me alone!"

  Alternative: Is that really true? Always? Never?

  "Everybody is giving me shit!"

  Alternative: A few people are trying to anger me, but most are not.

- *Name-calling triggers:* These are thought triggers that label a person as something, and they are often unkind, obscene, and designed to increase anger.

  "That son of a bitch (jerk, ass, etc.)!"

  She is not a _____, just a person I have a disagreement with.

4. At the end of this meeting, go around the group and ask each member to anticipate a possible "anger trigger" situation that may arise before the next meeting. If time permits, role-play a behavioral rehearsal of that anticipated situation, using the self-control techniques learned to date.

COMPREHENSION CHECK DECISION POINT

(Proceed to next training element or remain for additional work.)

1. Anger trigger
2. Thought trigger

Attribution Awareness

This is an exercise to assist the students in understanding the problems that accompany misattribution of intent. The goal of the exercise is to make the students aware of possible biases in their evaluations of others' behavior and to help them reduce the impulsive urge to retaliate based on those biased cognitions (see Trainers' Hint III.5).

1. Obtain a general understanding of the words "intention" and "hostile." When one knows another's intention, what does that mean? When someone's intention is "hostile," what does that mean? Obtain concrete examples from the group members.

2. Discuss how intentions can be misread and provide a personal example (e.g., "I intended to pick up my friend on time, but the traffic was snarled due to an accident. My friend thought I intended to make him wait and was angry when I

arrived"). Ask students for their own examples of how someone else misread their intentions.

3. Trainers should read the first part of each of the following incidents. The group members should then decide individually what two possible intentions of the interaction were. (Possible responses are included for trainers; change the gender as required).

a. Robert was getting dressed after gym. When he turned around from his locker, he saw that his new Nikes were being carried away by a new kid named Eddie. Robert yelled at him, "Hey, man! Gimme back my shoes!" Eddie's intent was:

Hostile: He was trying to steal Robert's shoes.

Accidental: Eddie turned around, looked at the shoes he was carrying, then smiled and pointed to his own pair, exactly the same, only two sizes larger, still lying under the bench. "Sorry," he said.

b. Mike was standing at his open locker talking to Tricia when Louis walked by and knocked Mike's locker closed. Mike yelled, "Hey, what are you doin', man?" Louis' intention was:

Hostile: He was trying to pick a fight with Mike.

Accidental: Louis turned and looked at him, surprised. "Oh, hey! I thought you were Jerry Turner. I'm sorry. His locker is right here somewhere, too. I wasn't even looking. We do that to sort of kid around with each other. I'm sorry, man."

c. Juan was walking down the hallway between classes when Sean and some of his buddies approached from the other direction. Sean knocked into Juan and sent his books to the floor. Sean's intention was:

Hostile: He was showing off for his buddies and trying to pick a fight.

Accidental: One of Sean's buddies playfully jostled Sean into Juan without meaning to do so.

4. Ask the students why it is important to correctly guess what someone else's intentions are (e.g., so you know how to respond; so you don't overreact; so you don't get angry for no reason and get in trouble). Hold a discussion about the ways that individuals can get information to help them determine what another's intentions are.

What are some ways that we can tell what a person's real intent is?

Trainers should encourage insights such as (1) looking for nonverbal cues, such as facial expressions and body posture, and (2) considering the context. How does a hostile facial expression look? How is that different from a surprised or embarrassed or playful facial expression? How does someone stand who is looking to be aggressive? How is that different from the body posture of someone who is being playful?

Are there differences among cultures? If the context up to this point has been playful, why would it suddenly turn hostile? (See Trainers Hint III.6).

5. Have the group members devise and role-play their own provocations. Player #1 should be provoked in some fashion (shoved, gestured at, books knocked over, etc.) by player #2. Player #1 should then say aloud, "STOP AND THINK," then take *one long calming breath*, and ascribe as many nonhostile—but realistic—intentions behind the alleged provocation as possible. For instance, STOP AND THINK (BREATH):

"Could be an accident. I'll wait and see."
"Maybe he's just playin'."
"Is he confusing me with someone else?"
"We've been cool up to now. He can't mean it."

Have the players replay their role plays with the provoker showing either aggressive or nonaggressive facial expressions or body postures that the other student must read accurately (see Trainers' Hint III.7).

COMPREHENSION CHECK DECISION POINT

(Proceed to next module or remain for additional work.)

1. Can student articulate a practical understanding of the terms "intention" and "hostile"?
2. Why is it important to consider alternative explanations for someone's behavior?
3. Can students demonstrate with evident understanding the use of the "stop and think" technique prior to ascribing intent?

MODULE IV

♦ ♦ ♦

Self-Instruction and Consequential Thinking

♦

Approximate number of meetings: Three to five

PREPARATION

Handout IV.1, "Reminders," copied for each group member
3″ × 5″ cards available

OUTCOMES

Knowledge Level

1. Students will understand that emotions can be influenced by direct cognitive self-statements.
2. Students will understand the use of self-instruction as a mechanism of anger regulation.
3. Students will be able to describe three temporal opportunities for the use of a self-instruction for anger regulation.
4. Students will understand how consequential thinking can help avoid undesirable problems in the school setting.

Skill Level

1. Students will be able to demonstrate anger regulation under practice conditions through the use of self-instruction.

FUNCTIONAL VOCABULARY

Reminders
Short-term consequences
Long-term consequences

COMMENT

Self-instruction as an approach to anger and other arousal-state management has been a widely researched subject for more than three decades (e.g., Meichenbaum, 1985; Novaco, 1975). Its value within a comprehensive program has been well established. The effectiveness of self-instruction is based on the premise that external events (name calling, pushing, taking of property) provoke anger only if these events are preceded, accompanied, or followed by self-statements of an anger-arousing nature. In other words, individuals must, in effect, tell themselves that it is time to become angry by way of applying anger-inducing meaning to the provocation. There is also research to suggest that individuals then maintain or escalate their anger states by labeling what they are feeling as anger (Novaco, 1975). In a similar way, individuals can learn to moderate or control their own anger by paying particular attention to how they choose to think about an anger-provoking event. In this module, students will learn a self-instruction technique referred to as "reminders" (Feindler & Ecton, 1986). This technique simply offers students a way to "self-instruct" or "self-coach" themselves through situations in which they have to try hard to keep from becoming aggressive.

TRAINERS' HINTS

Trainers' Hint IV.1

It is important for the trainers to continue to emphasize that anger control does not mean that you are *afraid* to show anger or *afraid* to fight. In some situations, those particular qualities may be maladaptive, even dangerous. Acknowledge to the students that you are aware that they often get double messages. Outside of school, within the peer culture, the student can get away with being more physical. Indeed, fighting prowess is a valued quality in many neighborhoods. However, regardless of what is adaptive in the neighborhood, when students enter the school building or the school bus, what may work in the neighborhoods is quickly punished. Fighting or other physical aggression as a means of problem solving is clearly not adaptive in school. Trainers should emphasize that anger control is designed to give students the ability to choose for themselves how they want to respond to an anger trigger. Remind the students that the more choices a person has to solve a problem, the more powerful that person becomes. Do not be afraid to acknowledge that fighting may be the safest option for a particular student in a particular situation. On the other hand, avoid being drawn in by the frequently heard protest, "You mean if some guy comes up and starts beating on you, you just stand there and get beat up?" All veteran school people know that fights don't happen that way. They are most often the result of extended transactions between individuals and often progress through many points at which the opportunities for nonviolent resolution are not recognized or are ignored.

Trainers' Hint IV.2

Some students may find the idea of "talking to yourself" socially embarrassing and may deny that they have any upcoming anger triggers. In such cases it is sometimes helpful to create a hypothetical situation in which the student is being pressured to become aggressive but in which it is very clearly in his or her best interest not to do so. "Let's say a teacher who you do not like starts giving you a hard time just as you are ready to get on the bus for the class trip to a local amusement park. In that circumstance, your thought triggers could get you so angry, you might lose it. What could you replace your thought triggers with that would give you more control? Further, let's say you knew ahead of time that this teacher would be there. How could you get yourself ready to manage yourself in the best possible way for you?"

Trainers' Hint IV.3

The skills rehearsal for the reminders technique has the potential for volatility and should be used only when the trainers can provide a safe environment for everyone. Students who do not yet have the requisite anger control to participate safely should be allowed to observe and provide feedback only. Trainers and students may feel more comfortable with an additional adult or two in the room, although care should be taken not to ramp up the anticipation for problems into a self-fulfilling prophecy. This activity was adapted from Larson and Lochman (2002). A substitute activity that does not involve taunting is included in this module.

Trainers' Hint IV.4

These rules were established so as not to create controversy in the school over allowing students to rehearse behaviors that would get them severely disciplined in the general environment and to provide some modicum of restraint on the activity. Trainers should vary from them only after very serious consideration. Students may ask which marginal words are allowed, and this is a reasonable discussion. Without obscenities, racial, or sexual slurs—the common verbal assault language of choice— many group members will struggle with effective taunts. Provide the taunters with time to think of some before putting them on the line. Ask: "If you wanted to trigger _____'s anger, what would you say to him (her)?" Additionally, the practicing student may have a personal sensitivity that he or she is not ready to be taunted about, and it is respectful to inquire about that ahead of time and prohibit it. If, however, this issue is a common anger trigger for the student, trainers may decide that at some point it will need to be addressed.

Trainers' Hint IV.5

Trainers should watch for the practicing student's potential to start "playing the dozens" or "slip fighting" with the taunters by returning taunts ("Oh, yeah? Well, your mother is . . . "). In such cases, stop the practice immediately, remind the student that he or she should be using only the reminders, and start over. Some may need multiple repetitions to overcome this well-rehearsed behavior. Additionally, trainers should stop the activity if the practicing student is having obvious difficulties and encourage to student to sit down and engage in anger reduction breathing.

Trainers' Hint IV.6

When a trainer asks the student who has been taunted to explain why he or she did not become angry under the taunting, one of them is very likely to say, "Because I knew this was just pretend. They didn't really mean it." Trainers should take that opportunity to praise the youth for the insight that, even if someone is saying cruel things about you, you do not have to become angry. The words have no magical power unless you believe that they do. In this case, the youth decided to believe that this was just pretend. Consequently, the words had no power, and anger was not a significant problem. Ask the students whether it would work as well when they are outside of the group if, instead of thinking a provocation was "pretend" they chose to believe that they, not the other person, had control of their own anger.

Trainers' Hint IV.7

The "Thinking Ahead" and other scenario activities often put students in situations in which, in real life, substantial peer pressure would argue mightily for an aggressive solution. Trainers should listen carefully for student responses in the group that are "socially acceptable" (what they think the trainers want to hear) but highly unlikely in the authentic setting. Challenge the students on those responses and help them to consider actions that would actually be acceptable to them. In some cases, delaying an aggressive response to another time ("I'd look for him after school") might be movement in a positive direction for a student with highly reactive aggression.

MODULE PROCEDURE

Reminders

1. Trainers should model a situation in which a high level of emotion needed to be moderated by self-instruction. For example:

> "When I was in college I had a job at a local department store. My boss was a great believer in the old adage that 'the customer is always right.' That meant no matter how rude or obnoxious the customers were, the salespeople always had to be pleasant and helpful. One day, a man came in to return a radio he said that he had purchased earlier. He didn't have the receipt, so I could not exchange it for him, and he started yelling at me. He called me 'stupid' and 'worthless' and a bunch of other names. I could feel my anger cues, but I knew that I would be fired if I got angry back at him, so I just kept saying to myself, 'Take it easy and smile. Take it easy and smile.' He finally yelled himself out and left. I kept my job."

Ask for student volunteers to model for the class exactly what they might say to themselves in the following situations:

a. It's the city championship basketball game; you are at the free throw line, down by one point, with one second left on the clock. You don't want to panic.
b. You are all alone, late at night in your home. You keep hearing odd noises downstairs—scraping, then a soft thumping noise, and then silence. You want to keep from becoming too frightened.
   - Point out that we often *remind* ourselves to stay calm in pressure situations by thinking through it.
   - Ask for other examples from the group members' experiences in which they were able to talk themselves out of becoming too nervous or frightened.
   - Tell the students, that just as we can remind ourselves to stay calm when we are nervous or frightened, we can also remind ourselves to stay calm when we are being provoked to anger.
   - Point out to the group that, just as some thought triggers can increase anger, other kinds of thoughts can decrease anger. Those anger-controlling thoughts are called "reminders" because they remind us that we can control our own anger.

2. Trainers should model their own use of *anger reducers plus reminders* that they use to help regulate their own anger intensity:

When I feel myself staring to become really angry at someone, I usually take a long, slow breath and say to myself _____.

3. Help the students understand that they can use reminders at different points in any potential anger problem situation (distribute Handout IV.1). Having an awareness of their own anger triggers in the school can help the students prepare for a potentially volatile encounter by using preparatory ("Before") reminders.

- Have each student identify a potential anger trigger situation that he or she will be encountering later that day or soon (e.g., problem class, person, or situation; see Trainers' Hint IV.2).
- Identify personally useful "Before" reminders that will help each student prepare for that encounter, or use the samples on the handout. This can be a chalkboard activity.
- Identify personally useful "During" reminders that will help each student manage his or her anger during that encounter. This can also be a chalkboard activity.
- Point out that timing is important when using the reminders technique. Remind students of how they can recognize their own cues for anger and that the proper time for using reminders is when they can feel their anger increasing.
- Remind students of the importance of the "After" phase, in which self-reinforcing or self-coaching occurs.

Reminders Skill Rehearsal (Important: see Trainers' Hint IV.3)

1. Have each group member decide on one or more "Before" and "During" reminders that are meaningful and useful to that person. Have each student write the reminders on a 3" × 5" card as an aid.

2. Point out to the students that just as practice is critical for athletic success, it is also critical for success when learning new personal skills.

"If you never shot a basketball in practice or never practiced dribbling a soccer ball, no one could ever expect you to do either in a real game situation. In the same way, if you don't have the opportunity to practice self-control in here, we can't expect you to do well out there. Today, we are going to practice."

3. Explain that the group will be working on controlling anger by using anger reducers and reminders in a situation of verbal harassment and taunting. One group

member at a time will volunteer to be taunted by the others. That group member will use the experience to practice the anger control techniques discussed so far.

4. Trainers should lay out two parallel tape lines on the floor, approximately 4 feet apart. The student who is practicing will stand behind one line, and the other group members will stand behind the second line. At the signal, the group members will taunt and verbally harass the practicing member for 30 seconds. Indicate that violating the line barriers will be cause for removal from the activity.

5. The taunters may use whatever verbal assaults they choose *except*:

a. They may not use racial or sexual slurs.
b. They may not use obscene language (see Trainers' Hint IV.4).

6. The practicing student should be granted 30 seconds to quietly repeat his or her "Before" reminder and to engage in long, slow breathing prior to the taunting.

7. At the signal, group members should begin their taunts. The practicing student should say his or her "During" reminders aloud in an audible voice. Reading from the card is permitted, but it must be read aloud (see Trainers Hint IV.5).

8. Trainers should signal the start and stop of both 30-second periods. They should subsequently encourage handshakes or high fives with the practicing student at the conclusion of each practice session and talk through any lingering interpersonal difficulties.

9. Trainers should debrief the practicing student at the conclusion of the practice session:

How did you do?
Why didn't you get furious at those remarks? (See Trainers' Hint IV.6.)
What can you differently next time to make improvements?
What would you need to do to show that sort of skill outside the group?

10. Modifications and additions to the reminders rehearsal include:

a. Trainers with self-concepts securely in place can model the practicing role first if there is confusion about what to do.
b. High-risk or reluctant students can be brought along slowly by starting with only the trainers doing the taunting, then progressing to the inclusion of additional group members one at a time.
c. Points can be awarded for a successful practice and for particularly helpful taunting behavior.
d. At the trainers' decision, students should transform the reminders from overt speech to covert self-instruction, either just mouthing them silently or thinking them.

11. Each group member should have at a minimum five to seven opportunities for practice in the group room context until both trainers and student agree that the skill is becoming solidified. Taunts should be varied and intensified within the parameters of the rules and safe training. This continued practice should be maintained even in the face of student protestations if the trainers believe it necessary.

12. Trainers should then vary the context by relocating to other areas of the building and continuing the practice (e.g., to the restroom, to the gym, to the locker area, etc.). Solicit locations and scenarios from the group members that reflect their legitimate experiences. *Utmost care should be taken not to embarrass the group members in front of curious peers or adults or disrupt other school activities.*

13. It is highly recommended that sufficient time be left at the ends of these reminder rehearsal meetings for students to relax and de-escalate from the energy of the activity. Trainers may once again need to remind students about confidentiality agreements. As always, students who are upset or agitated should remain with the trainers for individual attention before being allowed to continue on to class.

Alternative or Additional Rehearsal Activity

This activity may be done in lieu of the taunting practice when trainers are concerned about safety, or it may be done in addition to it.

1. Trainers should have each student role-play scenes from their completed hassle logs, using the anger reducer plus reminders.

2. For the role-plays, start with overt speech reminders from the 3″ × 5″ cards, then progress to covert reminders.

3. Remember to allow only anger-control role plays; no "before and after" scenes.

4. Consider videotaping the role plays for playback and analysis. The use of videotape wherein the student is his or her own positive model can be a powerful training aid.

COMPREHENSION CHECK DECISION POINT

(Proceed to next training element or remain for additional work.)

1. Does the student have knowledge and skill with "Before" reminders?
2. Does the student have knowledge and skill with "During" reminders?
3. Does the student have knowledge and skill with "After" reminders?

Thinking Ahead

1. Trainers should introduce *thinking ahead* as another procedure to use in conflict or anger-provoking situations. Explain that thinking ahead is a self-instruction

problem-solving technique that helps the student to estimate ahead of time the possible consequences of excessive anger or aggression in a conflict situation. Thinking ahead uses the following contingency statement:

"*If* I (misbehave) now, *then* I will (future negative consequences)."

2. Trainers should model some examples of if–then thinking from their own experience. Ask students to volunteer incidents from their own experiences in which stopping to think things out first helped them to avoid negative consequences. Ask them to predict what might have happened had they not stopped to think first.

3. Explain to students that fighting is sometimes one of the consequences of not thinking ahead. Tell them that the group is now going to brainstorm two lists: (1) all the positive consequences of fighting and (2) all the negative consequences of fighting. Write this list on the chalkboard.

"Tell me all the positive things that you can think of that people get out of fighting in school? What good comes from choosing to fight in the classroom or on school grounds?"

Feel good (if you win)
Buddies think you're tough
Get even
People leave you alone

Note: Most positives have the proviso "if you win. . . . "

"Now tell me all the negative consequences of fighting. What bad things can come from choosing to fight?"

Get hurt or killed
Hurt or kill someone
Get sued
Get suspended or expelled
Bad reputation
Revenge cycle begins
Clothes ripped

The negative list will be longer than the positive.

4. Trainers should help students differentiate short- and long-term consequences, noting that most positives are short term. Emphasize that *reminders can*

give students the cool head needed to use thinking ahead, which will help get the best possible consequences.

5. On the chalkboard, write:

reminder + thinking ahead + positive behavior

6. For the following scenarios, ask each student to supply a response that will be in his or her best interest, using the "*If I . . . then. . . . So, I will . . .* " formulation of consequential thinking. The behavioral decision should be in the form of a positive or prosocial behavior, instead of just what the student will not do (see Trainer's Hint IV.7).

Example: "Be cool. *If I* shove him, *then* he's gonna come back at me. *So, I will* just tell him this ain't worth a suspension from school and walk off."

- A student asks you to let him hide his knife in your locker.
- A student sits in your usual desk in English class and tells you to find another.
- The math teacher accuses you wrongly of cheating on a test and gives you a pass to the office.
- The shop teacher makes a cruel and sarcastic remark about you.
- Some students want you to help them steal a computer from the lab.

7. Using the completed hassle logs or knowledge about actual upcoming trigger events, trainers should have each student role-play the use of thinking ahead to avoid negative consequences.

COMPREHENSION CHECK DECISION POINT

(Proceed to next training Module or remain for additional work.)

1. Can the students articulate the value of assessing short and long-term consequences?
2. Can the students demonstrate effective understanding of the process of thinking ahead with authentic, current concerns?

MODULE V

◆ ◆ ◆

Social Problem-Solving

◆

Approximate number of meetings: Five to seven

PREPARATION

Handouts V.1, V.2, and V.3 copied for group members
Cards for "What Can I Do?" game prepared

OUTCOMES

Knowledge Level

1. Students will appreciate that difficult daily struggles can be usefully framed as structured problems to be solved.
2. Students will understand that problems can be defined in terms of personal goals and impeding obstacles.
3. Students will know the five sequential steps in a problem-solving process.
4. Students will appreciate the need to generate multiple possible solutions to difficult problems and to anticipate the consequences of each.
5. Students will understand a process for self-evaluation and self-coaching on problem-solving efforts.

Skill Level

1. Students will be able to reframe an existing problem into a goals-and-obstacles format.
2. Students will be able to generate multiple problem solutions and to provide and evaluate anticipated consequences for each solution.
3. Students will successfully address an authentic problem in the school setting using the stepwise problem-solving process.

FUNCTIONAL VOCABULARY

Goal
Obstacle
Anticipate

COMMENT

Module V addresses the training of problem-solving skills. This is a natural furthering of the skills taught in Modules I–IV, in which the students learned that they have the ability to exercise self-control in conflict situations. Learning to manage anger and aggression sets the stage for making decisions about the alternative methods that can be used to resolve interpersonal problems and conflicts. Even if a student can successfully demonstrate more effective self-control, that student still needs to be provided with additional tools for decision making. Problem solving typically is seen as a sequence of defining the problem, considering the alternatives, evaluating possible consequences of those alternatives, making a decision, and acting. Module V will take the students through this sequence.

One of the most prominent skill deficits that reactive–aggressive students have in common is a deficit in the quality and quantity of their problem-solving solutions (e.g., Lochman, Meyer, Rabiner, & White, 1991; Pepler, Craig, & Roberts, 1998). Whereas the great bulk of this research is with preadolescents, logic and experience argue for continued solution-generation difficulties into adolescence. The oft-heard rhetorical excuse of, "What else was I supposed to do?" after an aggressive incident exemplifies this learning deficit. Once students have had some experience with generating alternative solutions to problem situations, it is critical to give them a procedure that will lead them to the alternative that is in their best interest. Looking ahead and evaluating potential consequences is the most logical direction in which to take the process; however, many adolescents will need a great amount of structure to do this. The training in this module will build on the "thinking ahead" training addressed in Module IV.

Trainers should continue to emphasize and reinforce the use of the anger control skills addressed in the previous modules, even as the training now starts to focus on social problem solving. The skills are, of course, highly interrelated, and both are necessary for effective management of aggressive behavior. As noted earlier, the Think First training should not be approached in a purely lockstep manner. Rather, trainers should retain the flexibility to revisit previous skill elements as the needs of the students dictate, bearing in mind that no group of adolescents with high-risk behaviors is ever going to be completely skilled. Clinical judgment, flexibility, a reality focus, and a positive attitude need to rule the day.

TRAINERS' HINTS

Trainers' Hint V.1

Throughout this module, hypothetical problems will be offered for training. Although they are useful, generalization will be enhanced if the students are able to work with authentic problems that they are experiencing in the school, along with the hypothetical problems. As the meetings progress and more is learned about problem solving, it is recommended that the hassle logs be utilized liberally as contexts for learning the new skills.

Trainers' Hint V.2

Behavioral skills training is very frequently a useful aspect of anger and aggression management training. It is one thing to be able to generate and evaluate outcomes for potential responses to problem situations, but for many students, it is quite another to actually do them. It is often the case that the student can identify the most appropriate prosocial, nonaggressive behavior in the context of problem-solving training but that, from a skills standpoint, he or she does not know how to enact it. Trainers should attend to these potential training needs by carefully assessing the strengths and weaknesses of the group members in this area. For instance, if a group member identifies a behavior that calls for verbal assertion rather than aggression, trainers should insist that he or she demonstrate and practice that skill in the role play. Additionally, trainers may choose to access Goldstein and McGinnis (2000) for a comprehensive behavioral skills training program to augment the current training.

Trainers' Hint V.3

Some students can be motivated more effectively through the conveyance of a challenge or through bolstering their confidence. Meichenbaum (2001, p. 426) suggests the following language:

"This is going to take a lot of courage on your part. How will you begin?"
"Maybe it's too early to ask you to try doing. . . . "
"Like you said, it won't be easy."
"This is your chance to show others what you have learned."
"You have a difficult situation, but it sounds like you have the right idea."
"How confident are you (on a 0% to 100% scale) that you can do X?"

MODULE V PROCEDURE

Defining the Problem

1. Trainers should explain to students that the group is going to begin today to talk about making decisions. Observe that already today, each group member has made many decisions. Inquire:

"What decisions have you made already today?" (what to wear, how to fix hair, what to eat, whether to come to school, etc.)

2. On the board, write the two words:
   Decision   *Problem*

Explain that individuals make countless decisions on what to do and how to behave all day and most are relatively easy. A decision becomes a problem when one is not sure about what to do, about what decision to make. On the board, write the following equation:

GOALS + OBSTACLES = PROBLEM

Point out that all problems have two characteristics in common: a goal, that is, something we want; and one or more obstacles, or something that gets in the way of what we want.

Trainers should ensure a general understanding of the meaning of "obstacle" as pertaining not only to physical barriers but also to any circumstance that stands in the way of goal attainment. Propose the following to the group:

- Imagine that one's goal is to travel down a particular road to get to a friend's house, but a tree has fallen in the path. What is the obstacle?
- Imagine that a student's goal is to get a passing grade in algebra, but the student doesn't understand what the teacher is talking about. What is the obstacle? (lack of academic skill; not knowing how to seek help)
- Imagine that a student's goal is to make it to every class this week, but his or her friends want to skip Thursday after lunch. What is the obstacle? (loyalty to friends; lack of assertiveness skills).

3. Explain that solving a problem is easiest if it is approached one step at a time (distribute Handout V.1, "Stop and Think"):

Stop and Think: What Is the Problem?
What can I do?
What will happen if?
Which should I choose?
Now do it!
How did I do?

- The first step is to *stop and think* and decide just exactly what the problem is. The important point to stress here is that if a student has a problem, the student has to consciously *stop and think* or risk responding impulsively.
- Example: Suppose that you are working hard to keep out of trouble in school. Some friends stop you in the hallway between classes and want you to help them hassle and intimidate a much-disliked student in the rest room.
- What might the consequences be if you joined them without stopping to think about it? (Victim might tell; victim might get really hurt; a teacher could come in and catch us.)
- What if you stopped for moment first: How could you define this problem in terms of goals and obstacles? Solicit responses.

> I am trying to stay out of trouble in school (the goal), but I want to keep my friends (obstacle).

Trainers should point out that saying to oneself "stop and think" will help give a student time to decide what to do. The words "stop and think" are much like a reminder that we learned about earlier. We are once again "reminding" ourselves not to act without defining the problem first.

4. Trainers should have the group define this problem (change pronoun gender as desired):

"Imagine that you are about to go into school. Just before you go inside, your cousin comes up to you and begs you to leave school with him to go look for some kids who were threatening him earlier on the way to school. You have two very important tests first and second period, and you are sure you can pass them. But he's your cousin and if he goes alone, he could get hurt. Stop and think: What is the problem?"

Students should define the problem: What are some possible *goals* and what are the *obstacles* to those goals? Write them on the chalkboard.

5. Trainers should have the students think about and define a problem that is current in their lives and frame it in terms of their goals and the obstacles preventing them from easily reaching those goals. School problems are desirable, but social and family problems are allowed to in order to help teach this construct. A useful way of framing this exercise is to have the problems stated in the format: "I want . . . but . . ." with the BUT introducing the obstacle (e.g., "I want my little brother to stay out of my room, but my mother always takes his side").

Trainers should emphasize the importance of "I" statements in problem definition. In other words, the goal must be owned by the individual, because from a practical standpoint, the only behavior one can change for certain is one's own. Trainers should emphasize that it does little good to say that *your* problem will be solved when *someone else* decides to change his or her behavior. For example, "This group of kids is always hassling me" is not a problem statement; it is only a statement of fact. If one adds the goal statement prefix, "I want to stay out of trouble but . . . ," the problem is stated, and it opens up the possibility for potential solutions (see Trainers' Hint V.1).

COMPREHENSION CHECK DECISION POINT

(Proceed to next training element or remain for additional work.)

1. Do the students understand the relationship between goals and obstacles?
2. Can the students create a problem definition consisting of personal goals and evident obstacles?

What Can I Do?: Introduction to Alternative Solutions

1. Trainers should tell the students that today they are going to talk about and practice the second step in effective problem solving, which is answering the question, "What can I do?" Explain that, too often, when confronted with a tough problem, we all simply go ahead and try to solve it with the first thing that pops into our heads. Note that this method often works for common, easy decisions but that as the problems get more complicated, picking the wrong solution can create even bigger problems.

2. Trainers should model an incident from their own experience in which they resisted doing the first thing that came to mind and considered a better alternative.

3. Ask students: "What would you do if you were put in charge of deciding (select one)":

- What new car your family should buy?
- What music to play at the homecoming dance?
- Where the class trip should be?

4. After this discussion, provide the students with Handout V.2, "Finding Alternative Solutions," and continue with additional discussion, addressing the usefulness of the suggestions on the handout to the problems in Step 3.

5. Play the "What Can I Do?" Game. Trainers should divide the students into suitable groups of two to three students per group. To each group, trainers should distribute three 3″ × 5″ problem cards, chosen from the following problem list. Make certain each group gets the same three problems. Have each group choose a recorder who will do the writing and speaking for the group.

Say:

> "This is called the 'What Can I Do?' game. The object of the game is to come up with as many possible solutions to the problems on the card as you can. We call this 'brainstorming.' The only rule is that the solution must be *possible*; that is, you may not use magic, silly, or otherwise impossible alternatives. I will be the final judge of whether a solution is truly possible and serious. Remember: the solutions only have to be possible and serious, they do not have to good, lawful, or even smart."

- The goal of this game is to get students to realize that most problems have multiple possible solutions. Trainers should allow the students as much time as needed or, if preferred, set a timer for added fun.
- When all the distributed problems have been "brainstormed," have the recorder stand and read their group's solutions. Dismiss the silly or impossible solutions, and keep a total for each group on each problem on the board.
- Play the game repeatedly, mixing the groups and changing the problems. Trainers should devote two or more meetings to this activity and should feel free to come up with other, locally relevant problems.

Problem List

1. A stranger (student) bumps into you in the hall.
2. A gym teacher picks on you and makes you do extra pushups almost every day.
3. You see a stranger (student) trying to open your locker.
4. A group of older kids threaten to beat you up after school.
5. You are eating lunch and a student you don't like walks by and whispers, "Punk."
6. A kid you sort of know wants you to hold some drugs in your locker; he offers drugs or money in return.
7. Another student makes an insulting remark about your mother while the two of you are getting dressed after gym.

8. You are cutting class, and, down the hall, a teacher you don't know yells at you to stop and wait.
9. Your friend is upset and shoves you at your locker because you dissed him in front of the class.
10. You copied someone's homework, got busted, and you know who told on you.
11. A teacher accuses you wrongly of writing a gang symbol on the bathroom wall.
12. A friend comes by school with a car he stole and suggests you go for a ride with him.
13. Another student dumps your milk over at lunch. You think maybe it was on purpose.
14. You start your math homework but get stuck on the first problem.
15. Your girlfriend/boyfriend offers you a joint outside before school.
16. You need more money, your parents won't give it to you, and you are too young for a work permit.
17. You are studying for a final exam. A friend wants you to go to a concert instead.
18. You're not sure, but you think this particular student is spreading a false rumor about you.
19. You feel hopelessly lost in math or algebra class.
20. It's the first nice day of spring; your friends want to skip, but you have two tests to take.
21. Your girlfriend/boyfriend breaks up with you. You feel miserable.
22. Your mother forbids you to see a friend again.
23. In science class, the two kids beside you were talking. The teacher blames you and tells you to get out.
24. You get an F on your report card in English, but you are sure that you earned a C.
25. Instead of going out with your friend, you worked hard on your homework. Now he wants to copy it in study hall.

What Will Happen If . . . ?: Anticipating Consequences

1. Trainers should assist the group toward an understanding of the word "anticipate." Related words include: "predict," "expect," "foresee." Trainers should point out that learning how to anticipate what will happen when we choose to do something gives us power over what happens to us.

2. Trainers should engage the students in an anticipation exercise. Require the students to be as specific as possible in their responses. Do not accept, "You'll get in trouble." Have the students describe exactly what the "trouble" will be to the extent possible.

(Ask) "What if you were stopped by a teacher in the hallway after the bell rang. Look at your choices of behavior and tell me what is most likely to happen if . . ."

1. You run off?
2. You ignore the teacher and keep walking?
3. You explain your tardiness respectfully?
4. You call the teacher a name?
5. You shove the teacher?

(Ask) "*What if a student next to you in class calls you a dirty name under his breath so no one but you heard him? What will most likely happen if . . .*"

1. You stand up and shove him over?
2. You control your anger during class and beat him up in the hall afterward?
3. You control your anger and ignore him?
4. You control your anger and try to resolve the problem later?

3. Write on the board and point out to students that one of the best ways of looking at possible consequences is to ask:

If I do (this):
What is the *worst* that could probably happen?
What is *most likely* to happen?

4. Trainers should select some sample problem situations from the problem list for the "What Can I Do?" game (and/or have students generate their own) and for each alternative solution or response to the problem, have students apply the two consequence questions just given. For example:

Question 3. You see a stranger (student) trying to open your locker.
    Alternative 1: Run up, slam him into the locker, and kick his butt.
        What is the *worst* that could probably happen?
          You could hurt him badly and have legal trouble
        What is *most likely* to happen?
          Some teacher will see and you're off to the office.
    Alternative 2: Watch from a distance to see if he's really trying or at the wrong locker. If he continues, then confront him verbally.
        What is the *worst* that could probably happen?
          He might take a swing at you.
        What is *most likely* to happen?
          He gives you some b.s. story and gets scared.

5. Trainers should now have students role-play selected problems from the problem list. Students should rotate turns as the identified problem solver while the others play supporting roles. Each problem-solver should proceed through the steps for problem solving aloud, including (1) defining problem, (2) generating alternatives, and (3) anticipating consequences. Allow them to use Handout V.1 as an aid. *Each student should have multiple opportunities as the problem-solver.* Trainers should encourage realism!

COMPREHENSION CHECK DECISION POINT

(Proceed to next training element or remain for additional work.)

1. Can the students articulate the value of generating alternative responses to problem situations?
2. Can the students articulate two or more techniques for generating alternative responses to problem situations?
3. Can the students demonstrate through role-play a functional understanding of the first three steps of the problem-solving process?

What Will I Do?: Selecting and Enacting Problem-Solving Behavior

1. Now that students are gaining skill at anticipating and evaluating the consequences of their choices, trainers should point out that deciding which choice is best is the next step. Often, this decision will come more easily if the first three steps have been followed. Use these two examples or use authentic problems from the students' own current experiences. Have each student go through the first *four steps* in a realistic role-play of the incidents, using the overt or think-aloud procedure, including a decision about what they will do at the "Now Do It!" step:

a. Almost every day in your English class, your teacher says to you, "Why do you even bother coming? You're going fail this class anyway."
b. A student next to you in class calls you a dirty name under his breath so no one but you heard him.

- Remember, a student cannot perform a skill that he or she does not know how to do. For example, one cannot be assertive rather than aggressive if one does not know how to be assertive first (see Trainers Hint V.2).
- At the "Now Do It!" step, students should assess their own skill capacities and their needs for additional environmental supports in order to make their selected response work. Trainers should query the students at this step. For example:

"Do you know how to do that? How could you learn?"

"How would you do that? Show me."

"What do you mean by _____? What does that behavior look like?"

"When or where have you done similar behavior? Did it work then?"

"Is there someone in the school who could help you do that? How could that person help?"

3. Trainers should distribute Handout V.3, "Problem-Solving Worksheet." Students should now decide on a current school-based problem that they will address and work it out in writing on the worksheet. Trainers should facilitate, but attend carefully to individual skill levels for this juncture of the training. Students who are still struggling with understanding one or more of the steps should be identified and provided with additional opportunities for learning.

- Is the problem defined usefully, with goals and obstacles clearly stated?
- Are there at least two reasonable alternative solutions proposed?
- Are the anticipated consequences for each solution reality based?
- Is the proposed solution behavior well defined and within the current skill base of the student? Are needed supports available?

4. Trainers should now challenge the group members to actually engage in the problem-solving process that they have proposed on the worksheet and report their experiences at the next meeting (see Trainers' Hint V.3). Trainers should continue this exercise in subsequent meetings as long as it proves useful.

How Did I Do?: Self-Evaluation and Self-Coaching

1. Trainers should point out that it is always helpful to take some time to look carefully at the choice you made in a problem situation. Whether one is pleased with the consequences or not pleased, it is important to take some time to look back. Have the students ask themselves (trainers should write the following on the chalkboard):

- "Did I make the right choice?"
- "If so, nice job!"
- "If not, why?"
- "What should I do differently next time?"

2. At this juncture, it is important for trainers to discuss the issue of what happens if the students try to apply what they have learned but still get in trouble. Students will frequently report back that, "I tried, but this stuff don't work." The likelihood is high that historically aggressive or problematic adolescents are going to

continue to be that way out of sheer habit, at least in the short term. Emphasize that there is no magic in the program or any of techniques for anger control or problem solving that have been discussed:

> "As with learning any new skill, you have to practice. And as with any new skill, you will not be perfect the first time or every time thereafter. How many here made the first basket they ever shot? How many now hit them *every* time without ever missing? In the same way, learning new ways of coping with anger and aggression and solving tough problems takes time and practice. And you won't always do it right. Mistakes are a part of life."

Provide students with model self-statements for coping with failure. For example:

- "I messed up, but I know why."
- "I won't make the same mistake twice."
- "I need to look at consequences more carefully."
- "Nobody's perfect. I'll do better next time."

3. Ask for suggestions from the students as to what kinds of self-coping statements they can say to themselves if they make some mistakes.

MODULE V ADDENDUM: FOLLOW-UP AND PROGRESS MONITORING

Booster Meetings

It is important to avoid the tendency to "finalize" the training as if it was a fixed curriculum that has been completed. Rather, once the training elements in Module V have been sufficiently addressed, trainers should assess the current competency levels of the students and make determinations about what should be next and how frequently the meetings need to occur. It is highly likely that, at some later point in the year, after the skills in Module V have been trained, the meeting frequency can be reduced to every other week. These "booster" meetings should continue active skill training and support, addressing current concerns, problem-solving new strategies, and shoring up weak training elements. Reinstituting the previous meeting frequency should always remain an option.

Trainers should continue the collaborative mentorship relationship by actively soliciting input from the students about challenges they are facing and issues on which they want to work. They are not "cured" in any sense of the term; rather, they now possess a set of helpful insights and emerging skills that will need continuous nourishment and support from all of the support personnel and trainers. Indeed, the likelihood is great that, for some of the students, behavioral skills training will need to be an expected—and accepted—feature of their experience in the school setting for the years to come.

Progress Monitoring

Those who have worked with high-risk adolescents have heard the refrain, "I don't think all your counseling did him any good. He's still one of the biggest problems in the school." My response, sometimes expressed or sometimes just politely thought, is: "Yes, but how much more of a problem would he be if he hadn't been working so hard with my group all this time?" That is a reasonable question, and it needs to be kept in mind as trainers assess the progress and outcomes of their efforts. Where are the data that will demonstrate that measurable gains have been made by some or all of the group members? Bear in mind that the purpose of the outcome data gathering proposed here is to help document clinical usefulness and inform the trainers' efforts at intervention modification, not for publication in a research journal. As a general rule with data such as these, it is most advantageous to look for individual positive trends rather than "significant" differences across time.

1. *Official school records.* Trainers should graph official school data that were collected on each student at the outset and (one hopes) subsequently maintained as the group progressed. These sources may include disciplinary information such as number of office referrals, number of detentions, and number of suspensions in or out of the school. Disciplinary categories may be further subdivided into aggressive and nonaggressive violations or other subdivisions that may reflect the problems faced by a particular student. As an example, a graph of the number of office referrals received by Kevin shows a slight downward trend over the course of the weekly training sessions. If the graph is adjusted to reflect only those office referrals for anger- or aggression-related offenses, the downward trend is more pronounced.

When trainers are examining official school records over time to look for trends, it is important to bear in mind that *time itself* is a major explanatory variable for change. Veteran school professionals understand that the school year has rhythms of high and low problem times, often related to the relative weeks before and after an extended vacation time or, in northern areas, the changes in seasons. Consequently, when examining behavioral trend data for Think First group members, trainers should attempt to view the trend in the context of what the trends were for the rest of the school during that time period. In other words, imagine that Kevin had 12 office referrals in September and that the total number of office referrals for all students from his sixth-grade teaching team that month was 72. Then, after 2 months of intervention, Kevin's November office referral figure was only 6, but the total for the rest of the students in his sixth-grade team during this was only 40. Was it the intervention or something in the general school climate that was responsible for Kevin's apparent positive gain? Similarly, what if the rest of the cohort's discipline referrals increase in a given month, but Kevin's stays the same? Such an occurrence might be seen as positive, because Kevin's percentage of the total number of office referrals declined; he was bucking a trend. In other words, be careful of overinterpreting these sorts of data, but also be careful not to miss useful information that may be slightly hidden in the mix.

2. *Classroom Progress Monitoring Report Form.* The collected Classroom Progress Monitoring Report forms may be graphed for individual students along any of the 5 Likert-scaled items. For instance, trainers may be interested in any changes in the Vocal Disruptive Behavior item or the Self-Control of Anger item over time. Examining the trends on this form may allow the trainers to gather information useful in future academic planning regarding the classroom environmental context of problem behavior for particular individuals. For example, why were clear behavioral improvement trends seen in some classes but not others?

3. *Data from psychometric instruments.* Repeated administrations of any self-report measures or teacher checklists can provide additional information for trainers, particularly when looked at in the context of the convergence of multiple sources of data. Data from a single source, such as a lower overall score on the Multidimensional School Anger Inventory, may not be noteworthy when viewed in isolation. However, when this positive piece of information is added to other data sources, a converging trend may be readily observable. Trainers are urged to consider that the accumulation of multiple, same-directional trends, even minor ones, can present converging evidence that can be interpreted as clinically useful.

A caveat: In my experience I have found that using commercial teacher checklists as measures of treatment gain adds more confusion than clarity about a student, and I have come to devalue them in comparison with more authentic data. My hypothesis is that it may be difficult for teachers to get past the fact that Kevin exhibited the most problematic behavior in the class back in September and that now, in May, Kevin is still the most problematic. That highly salient teacher observation often clouds the additional fact that, although his relative position in the class may remain unchanged, he may have demonstrated undeniable gains on numerous measures of authentic progress. High-risk, externalizing students can make some teachers' lives miserable, and for many of them, it is difficult to be objective on behavior check sheets. I consider that to be more "human" than "unprofessional" and, consequently, rarely ask it of them. I believe that the biweekly Classroom Progress Monitoring Report, with its shorter, more frequent assessment periods, is a more reliable measure.

Appendices

◆

CURRENT BEHAVIOR SCREENING FORM

Student's Name _____ Date of Birth _____

Today's Date _____ Information is for the _____–_____school year

Informant's Name _____ Position _____

Behaviors observed in the current year:

1. Angry physical aggression (pushing, grabbing, scratching) against peers; not playful

0	1	2	3	4
Not observed	Once	2–5 times	6–10 times	Chronic behavior

2. Physical fighting with peers; punches thrown

0	1	2	3	4
Not observed	Once	2–5 times	6–10 times	Chronic behavior

3. Angry *threats* of physical aggression against peers

0	1	2	3	4
Not observed	Once	2–5 times	6–10 times	Chronic behavior

4. Outbursts of temper resulting in destroyed peer or own property

0	1	2	3	4
Not observed	Once	2–5 times	6–10 times	Chronic behavior

5. Angry physical aggression (pushing, grabbing, scratching) against adults

0	1	2	3	4
Not observed	Once	2–5 times	6–10 times	Chronic behavior

6. Angry *threats* of physical aggression against adults

0	1	2	3	4
Not observed	Once	2–5 times	6–10 times	Chronic behavior

7. Angry *threats* with an implement (e.g., stick, bat, scissors)

0	1	2	3	4
Not observed	Once	2–5 times	6–10 times	Chronic behavior

8. Physical aggression with an implement (e.g., stick, bat, scissors)

0	1	2	3	4
Not observed	Once	2–5 times	6–10 times	Chronic behavior

(continued)

9. Angry destruction of school property

0	1	2	3	4
Not observed	Once	2–5 times	6–10 times	Chronic behavior

10. Other (Describe):

	1	2	3	4
	Once	2–5 times	6–10 times	Chronic behavior

Circle number of each intervention implemented in this current year:

1. School-based anger management skills training
2. Community-based anger management skills training
3. Other counseling (Type): _____
4. Classroom or school-wide behavior modification strategies
5. Behavioral contracting
6. Modified school day
7. Other (Describe):

Which positive behavioral supports were found to be most effective?

What insights and skills do teachers need to have to work most effectively with this student?

Contact information for follow-up:

Classroom teacher   Phone   E-mail

_____   _____   _____

Other _____   _____   _____

Other _____   _____   _____

INTERVENTION RECORD REVIEW

Reviewer _____ Date of Review _____

Student's Name _____ Date of Birth _____

Grade _____ Units Earned (H.S. only) _____ Homeroom _____

I. Office Referrals/Disciplinary Record

From _____ to _____ there have been _____ office referrals

Number:

___ Abusive Language   ___ Conduct   ___ Disobeying Authority   ___ Disrespect

___ Fighting   ___ Leaving without Permission   ___ Threatening   ___ Other

Temporal Pattern?

Setting Pattern?

Referral Source Pattern?

Notes:

II. Previous Behavioral Supports

Schoolwide Type(s):

Classroom Type(s):

Notes:

(continued)

III. Current Behavioral Supports

Schoolwide Type(s):

Classroom Type(s):

Notes:

IV. Previous Counseling/Skills Training

Dates and Locale:

____ None

Notes:

V. Academic Progress, Concerns, and Supports

High-Stakes Testing Status:

High School Units Earned ___ out of ___ Attempted

Current Grade Point Average _____

Apparent Academic Strengths _____

Apparent Academic Weaknesses _____

Current Academic Supports:

ADOLESCENT INTERVIEW

Student's Name _____   Interview Date _____

I. Problem Conceptualization

Tell me about how school is going for you these days.

Tell me about your school experience before this year.

What was the most serious problem you had before this year?

How did that problem turn out?

When was the last time you got in trouble/lost your temper/had a fight here in school?

Tell me about what happened with that.

Who is mostly responsible for the problems that you are having in school? Explain.

Tell me how you get along with your teachers. (Focus on any problem relationships.)

How do other kids add to the problems you have in school?

Tell me about how you are doing in your classes, grade-wise.

Best class? Why? What do *you do* that makes it successful? (Probe locus of control.)

Worst class? Why? What do *you do* that brings you down in there?

II. Problem Resolution Efforts

What was the most successful year you ever had in school? Why? (Probe for supports.)

How would you change your school day so that the serious problems wouldn't happen?

What happens when you lose your temper with another student?

How do you control your temper when you want to? Does this work all the time?

What do teachers do to help you control your temper? To make it worse?

What have teachers or others done to help you to avoid problems in the past?

What sorts of things have worked best to help you avoid problems in school?

Have you ever had counseling, in school or out? Tell me about it. How did it help?

(continued)

III. Willingness for Skills Training

Before the student leaves the interview session, secure a verbal commitment to attend the first group meeting.

> "I am planning to run a counseling group here in school. All of the participants in the group will be students such as you who have been having serious problems getting along with others in this building. All the participants will be students who absolutely need to develop new skills for managing their anger and their aggression if they want to succeed in school. I believe strongly that you will benefit from working with me and the others in this group. We will meet once per week for the entire semester. In this group, we will learn skills for controlling anger in tough situations around the school, how to set and meet personal goals, and how to solve difficult problems with other people, including teachers, administrators, and other students. I will explain more about it at our first meeting, and you can hold off on your final decision until then. However, from what you do know, will you be willing to consider participating? Our first meeting will be _____, and I will remind you and make sure you have a pass. Can I answer any other questions for you?"

BRIEF PROBLEM ASSESSMENT INTERVIEW

Teacher/Administrator: _____ Student: _____ Date: _____

I. Behavior Summary

1. General Description of Aggressive Behavior:

2. Behavior Setting
   (A precise description of the time and settings in which the problem behaviors
   occur; e.g., *"When and where does _____ do this?"*)

3. Identify Antecedents/Triggering Events
   (What is typically happening right before the problem behavior occurs? e.g., class
   transitions, peer teasing, etc.)

   (Is there anything about the individual's internal state—physical well-being,
   emotional condition - that is related to the occurrence of the problem? This could
   be related to medication, sleep, etc.)

4. Identify Consequences
   (What happens after the problem behavior has occurred?, e.g., "What do you do
   when _____ starts to get angry and loud? What do the other students do?")

   Interviewee does:

(continued)

Others do:

5. Behavior Frequency
   (*How often do you see this behavior?*)

6. What Are the Conditions Under Which This Behavior Is Least Likely To Be Observed? (e.g., during gym, during supervised seatwork, when _____ is absent, etc.)

   What Is It about These Conditions That Helps?

7. Teacher/Administrator Attribution for the Behavior:
   (*e.g., "What do you think sets _____ off like that?"*)

II. Function and Replacement Behavior

8. Needs/Functions. What function or purpose does the behavior seem to serve for the student? What need is being expressed by the behavior?

   <u>Escape</u>

   - Avoid demand or request
   - Avoid an activity/task
   - Avoid a person
   - Escape the setting
   - Other _____

   <u>Communicate/Acquire</u>

   - Express anger
   - Gain adult attention
   - Gain peer attention/approval
   - Get sent to preferred adult
   - Other _____

9. Skill Deficits. What does the student need to know and be able to do to avoid this problem?

CLASSROOM PROGRESS MONITORING REPORT

Student's Name _____ Teacher _____

Subject _____ Period _____

For the week _____ to _____

Please consider the week as a whole.

1. Adherence to classroom rules and routines

Above the class average	At the class average	Below the class average	Well below class average
4	3	2	1

Optional Comment:

2. Vocal disruptive behavior

Above the class average	At the class average	Below the class average	Well below class average
4	3	2	1

Optional Comment:

3. Self-control of anger

Above the class average	At the class average	Below the class average	Well below class average
4	3	2	1

Optional Comment:

4. Homework returned

Above the class average	At the class average	Below the class average	Well below class average
4	3	2	1

Optional Comment:

(continued)

5. In-class assignment effort

Above the class average	At the class average	Below the class average	Well below class average
4	3	2	1

Comment:

6. (other) _____

Above the class average	At the class average	Below the class average	Well below class average
4	3	2	1

Comment:

_____

Teacher signature

Please return to _____

MULTIDIMENSIONAL SCHOOL ANGER INVENTORY

Name _____ Age _____ Grade _____

School _____ Date of Birth ___/___/___

These pages ask about some of the feelings, ideas, and behaviors you may have at school. Give an answer to each number (1–54). Respond by filling in the number that best shows your answer. Remember, there are no right or wrong answers.

If these things happened to you AT SCHOOL, how mad would you be?

1	2	3	4
I wouldn't be mad at all	I'd be a little angry	I'd be pretty angry	I would be furious

1. You didn't notice that someone put gum on your seat and you sit on it.	① ② ③ ④
2. At school, two bigger students take something of yours and play "keep away" from you.	① ② ③ ④
3. You tell the teacher that you're not feeling well but he or she doesn't believe you.	① ② ③ ④
4. Someone in your classroom acts up, so the whole class has to stay after school.	① ② ③ ④
5. You ask to go to the bathroom and the teacher says "no."	① ② ③ ④
6. You go to your locker in the morning and find out that someone has stolen some of your school supplies.	① ② ③ ④
7. Someone in your class tells the teacher on you for doing something.	① ② ③ ④
8. You get sent to the principal's office when other students are acting worse than you.	① ② ③ ④
9. The teacher's pet gets to do all of the special errands in class.	① ② ③ ④
10. Somebody cuts in front of you in the lunch line.	① ② ③ ④
11. You are trying to do you work in school and someone bumps your desk on purpose and you mess up.	① ② ③ ④
12. You study really hard for a test and still get a low grade.	① ② ③ ④
13. Somebody calls you a bad name.	① ② ③ ④

(continued)

Publically available at www.education.ucsb.edu/school-psychology/MSAI/PDF/MSAI-English.pdf

14. Someone starts a mean rumor about you that spreads all over the school.	① ② ③ ④
15. Someone steals a note that you are trying to pass to a friend.	① ② ③ ④
16. Someone tries to take away your boyfriend or girlfriend.	① ② ③ ④
17. You get cut from a team or club at school (for example, basketball, chorus, debate).	① ② ③ ④
18. Your best friend makes fun of your hair or clothes.	① ② ③ ④
19. A teacher gives a surprise quiz.	① ② ③ ④

Do you disagree or agree with these ideas?

1	2	3	4
Strongly Disagree	Disagree	Agree	Strongly Agree

20. School is worthless (junk).	① ② ③ ④
21. School is really boring.	① ② ③ ④
22. Grades at school are unfair.	① ② ③ ④
23. There is nothing worth learning at school.	① ② ③ ④
24. Rules at school are stupid.	① ② ③ ④
25. Adults at school don't care about students.	① ② ③ ④
26. In class, I let others know when they are wrong or get in my way.	① ② ③ ④
27. Sooner or later even best friends at school let you down.	① ② ③ ④
28. I don't need anybody's help at this school for anything.	① ② ③ ④
29. Most days I get ticked off at someone or by something at school.	① ② ③ ④
30. At this school, teachers go out of their way to help students in tough times.	① ② ③ ④
31. Nobody at school respects me.	① ② ③ ④
32. You can trust people at this school.	① ② ③ ④

When you get mad at school, what do you do?

1	2	3	4
Never	Occasionally	Often	Always

33. When I'm angry, I'll take it out on who ever is around.	① ② ③ ④
34. I talk it over with another person when I'm upset.	① ② ③ ④
35. When I get angry, I think about something else.	① ② ③ ④
36. When I'm mad, I hate the world.	① ② ③ ④
37. When I get mad at school, I share my feelings.	① ② ③ ④
38. When I'm mad, I break things.	① ② ③ ④
39. Before I explode, I try to understand why this happened to me.	① ② ③ ④

(continued)

40. When I'm upset, I calm myself down by reading, writing, painting, or some similar activity.	① ② ③ ④
41. I get so mad that I want to hurt myself.	① ② ③ ④
42. If something makes me mad, I try to find something funny about it.	① ② ③ ④
43. When I'm mad, I let my feelings out by some type of physical activity like running, playing, etc.	① ② ③ ④
44. If I get mad, I'll throw a tantrum.	① ② ③ ④
45. I cry when I'm angry.	① ② ③ ④
46. When I'm angry, I want people to leave me alone.	① ② ③ ④
47 When I get mad my stomach or head aches.	① ② ③ ④
48. When I'm angry, I cover it up by smiling or pretending I'm not mad.	① ② ③ ④
49. When I'm mad at someone, I ignore them.	① ② ③ ④
50. When I'm angry, I want to be by myself.	① ② ③ ④
51. I punch something when I'm angry.	① ② ③ ④
52. When I get a bad grade, I figure out ways to get back at the teacher.	① ② ③ ④
53. When I'm mad at a teacher, I make jokes in class to get my friends laughing.	① ② ③ ④
54. When I get a bad grade on a test, I rip the test paper into little pieces.	① ② ③ ④

Thank you.

For more information: Michael Furlong, UCSB, Gevirtz School of Education, Center for School-Based Youth Development, Santa Barbara, CA 93016; *mfurlong@education.ucsb.edu; www.education.ucsb.edu/c4sbyd.*

SAMPLE PARENTAL CONSENT LETTER

Dear Parent/Guardian:

Your student, _____, is being asked to take part in a small counseling group. Your student is being asked to take part in this group because his teachers and I believe that it will help him/her in one or more of these goals we have for the group:

1. To learn how to improve control of anger or temper
2. To learn how to improve behavior and academic achievement in school
3. To learn how to improve problem-solving skills

The group will meet here at school once per week for about 25 weeks. We will meet on **(day).** The group leader(s) in charge will be **(name and title).** He/She/I can be reached at **(phone number.)**

In the group, the students will use role-playing and discussion to learn important anger control skills, how avoid negative confrontations with others, and how to solve problems with other students or adults. Careful attention to the student's academic progress will be maintained. A full explanation of each activity is available by calling the group leader at the number above. Please call if you have questions or to arrange a meeting here at school. Your support is very important. If, however, you decide that you do not want your student to participate, please know that we will continue to work with him/her in the classroom to the best of our ability. The school may be able to direct you to similar services in the community, if you prefer.

There are no foreseeable risks associated with participation in this group. Every effort will be made to see that your student misses as little classroom instruction as possible. The teachers will see to it that makeup time is made available, if needed.

Your student and his/her teachers may be asked to complete a behavior checklist so that the group leader can better help him/her in the group. The results will be kept confidential, although as the legal guardian, you may be able to inspect them or obtain a copy. The checklists that will be used are:

_____   _____

Please sign and return the tear-off form below. Keep the top for your files.

Sincerely,

(Name/Title)

(continued)

_____

....

(Check one)

____   I give my permission for my child, _____ to take part in the counseling group described above.

____   I do NOT give my permission.

_____   _____

Signature   Date

CARTA DE CONSENTIMIENTO DE PADRES

Estimados padres/tutores:

Su hijo, _____, ha sido seleccionado para tomar parte en un pequeño grupo de terapia. Su hijo ha sido seleccionado para tomar parte de este grupo porque su maestro(a) y yo consideramos que esto le ayudará en uno ó más de estas metas que son fijadas para el grupo:

1. aprender a controlar mejor sus enojos y reacciones negativas
2. aprender a mejorar la conducta y éxito académico en la escuela
3. aprender a mejorar las habilidades para resolver/solucionar conflictos

El grupo se reunirá en la escuela un día cada semana por aproximadamente 25 semanas. Nos reuniremos los _____. El encargado del grupo será _____. Se puede comunicarse por teléfono _____.

En el grupo, los niños utilizarán interpretaciones de papeles y discusiones para aprender las habilidades importantes de controlar los enojos, cómo evitar conflictos negativos con otros, y cómo resolver/solucionar los conflictos con otros estudiantes y adultos. El progreso académico del estudiante será vigilado cuidadosamente. Una explicación completa de cada actividad estará a su disposición con sólo llamar al número de teléfono antes mencionado. Por favor, llamen si tengan alguna pregunta o si desean hacer una cita en la escuela. Su cooperación es muy importante. Si por alguna razón ustedes decidieran que su niño no participe en el grupo, nosotros seguiremos trabajando con él en el salón de clases para que pueda ser un buen estudiante. La escuela se puede dirigir a servicios similares a éste que se encuentran en la comunidad, si prefieren.

No hay riesgos previsibles asociados con participación en este grupo. Se hará todo el esfuerzo posible para que el niño no pierda mucho tiempo de instrucción de clase. Su maestro(a) le dará tiempo adicional para terminar los trabajos, si fuera necesario.

Su hijo y su maestro(a) pueden ser contactos para completar un formulario para que el encargado del grupo pueda ayudar mejor a su hijo. Los resultados de estos formularios serán guardados confidencialmente, aunque ustedes como padres/tutores tienen la libertad de verlos si desean. Los formularios que se utilizarán son:

_____   _____

Por favor, firmen y devuelvan el talonario que se encuentra al final de ésta carta. Conserven la parte de arriba de éste carta para su información.

Sinceramente,

(continued)

_____

....

(Escoja uno)

____   Yo autorizo a mi hijo, _____, para participar en el grupo de terapia descrito arriba.

____   Yo NO autorizo.

_____   _____

Firma   Fecha

GUIDELINES FOR GENERALIZATION SUPPORT PERSONS

Support Person _____ Student's Name _____

Thank you for agreeing to serve as a generalization-support person for the above-named student. Because of the critical need to promote transfer of training from the group meeting to the school environment, this is an essential component of the anger and aggression skills training program. The role you will serve is one of observation and feedback: Keep an eye on the student's behavior while in the normal course of your duties, and give the student useful feedback on it. Please make a mental note of your interactions for later communication to the group leaders.

- Issue a friendly greeting to the student at least once per day.
- Watch for situations or "triggers" that seem to precede angry behavior.
- Observe the student's anger and/or aggression control strategies (e.g., turns away, leaves area, is verbally assertive).
- Use discreet, positive feedback when you observe evident anger control efforts or other appropriate behavior (e.g., "I like the way you ignored Charles," or "Nice job staying out of that fracas earlier").
- Offer descriptive feedback when problems arise (e.g., "You let Chris push your buttons. How can you avoid that next time?").
- Occasionally inquire about progress in the group (e.g., "How're things going in Think First?" and when appropriate, "I hear you're working pretty hard").
- Relay positive feedback from other staff members.

The skills training group meets: Day _____ Time _____
Please leave phone messages for the group leader at Ext. _____
You may also contact me (e-mail, etc.) _____

Thank you once again for agreeing to serve in this important role.

_____
Group Leader

ACADEMIC SELF-MONITORING FORM

Name _____ Week of _____ to _____

Class: _____   Check all that apply this week:
    O No unexcused absences
    O All homework turned in
    O Asked questions
    O Positive comment to teacher
    O _____

Class: _____   Check all that apply this week:
    O No unexcused absences
    O All homework turned in
    O Asked questions
    O Positive comment to teacher
    O _____

Class: _____   Check all that apply this week:
    O No unexcused absences
    O All homework turned in
    O Asked questions
    O Positive comment to teacher
    O _____

Class: _____   Check all that apply this week:
    O No unexcused absences
    O All homework turned in
    O Asked questions
    O Positive comment to teacher
    O _____

Class: _____   Check all that apply this week:
    O No unexcused absences
    O All homework turned in
    O Asked questions
    O Positive comment to teacher
    O _____

(continued)

Class: _____ Check all that apply this week:

    O No unexcused absences
    O All homework turned in
    O Asked questions
    O Positive comment to teacher
    O _____

Class: _____ Check all that apply this week:

    O No unexcused absences
    O All homework turned in
    O Asked questions
    O Positive comment to teacher
    O _____

Circle the number that best describes your week:

Successful effort   Good effort, some mistakes   Poor effort, many mistakes

10   9   8   7   6   5   4   3   2   1

THINK FIRST TRAINING OUTCOMES

Module I Knowledge Level

1. Students will understand the purpose of the group and the reasons for their inclusion.
2. Students will understand the procedures and times for future meetings.
3. Students will understand the behavioral rules of the group and applicable point system.
4. Students will understand that most of the behaviors that they engage in are choice behaviors.
5. Students will understand the relationship between antecedent, behavior, and consequence.
6. Students will be able to articulate at least one prosocial reason for learning how to improve their own capacity for self-control in challenging situations.

Module II Knowledge Level

1. Students will know how to complete a hassle-log self-monitoring procedure.
2. Students will be able to provide a definition of anger.
3. Students will understand that an individual's anger level can be described on a continuum of intensity, from mild to very strong.
4. Students will understand that anger has a physiological aspect that can be self-perceived, monitored, and controlled.
5. Students will be able to describe their own physiological responses to increased anger levels.

Module II Skill Level

1. Students will be able to demonstrate one or more palliative anger reducers in the group setting.

Module III Knowledge Level

1. Students will be able to identify their most problematic direct (external) anger provocations within the school setting.
2. Students will understand the meaning of the term "thought trigger" and be able to differentiate it from the term "anger trigger."
3. Students will be able to describe how a thought trigger can contribute to anger escalation.
4. Students will be able to describe a variety of potential thought triggers.
5. Students will understand how ascribing intent inaccurately can lead to anger and aggression.
6. Students will be able to describe facial features and body postures associated with anger or hostility.

(continued)

Module III Skill Level

1. Students will be able to demonstrate understanding of anger cues and anger reducers in the context of their own hassle-log incidents.
2. Students will show an ability to evaluate the intent of a potential provocation through the use of a "stop and think" technique paired with an anger reducer.

Module IV Knowledge Level

1. Students will understand that emotions can be influenced by direct cognitive self-statements.
2. Students will understand the use of self-instruction as a mechanism of anger regulation;
3. Students will be able to describe three temporal opportunities for the use of self-instruction for anger regulation.
4. Students will understand how consequential thinking can help avoid undesirable problems in the school setting.

Module IV Skill Level

1. Students will be able to demonstrate anger regulation under practice conditions through the use of self-instruction.

Module V Knowledge Level

1. Students will appreciate that difficult daily struggles can be usefully framed as structured problems to be solved.
2. Students will understand that problems can be defined in terms of personal goals and impeding obstacles.
3. Students will know the five sequential steps in a problem-solving process;
4. Students will appreciate the need to generate multiple possible solutions to difficult problems and to anticipate the consequences of each.
5. Students will understand a process for self-evaluation and self-coaching on problem-solving efforts.

Module V Skill Level

1. Students will be able to reframe an existing problem into a goals-and-obstacles format.
2. Students will be able to generate multiple problem solutions and provide and evaluate anticipated consequences for each solution.
3. Students will successfully address an authentic problem in the school setting using the stepwise problem-solving process.

Handouts

◆

BEHAVIOR A-B-C'S

A—Something Happens

B—What I Choose to Do

C—What Are the Consequences?

HASSLE LOG

Name _____ Date _____

Where was I?

____In class   ____In the gym

____In the hall   ____In the lunchroom

____In the rest room ____By my locker   ____(Where?) _____

What happened?

____Someone hit or pushed me   ____Someone took something of mine

____Someone provoked me   ____Someone showed me disrespect

____Someone said something   _____

What did I do?

____Used anger control   ____Hit or pushed them

____Walked away, left   ____(Other) ____

____Was verbally aggressive

How angry was I? (Circle Number)

Furious!	Pretty Upset	Irritated	Annoyed, but okay
10 9 8	7 6 5	4 3	2 1

How did I handle myself?

____Great! I controlled my anger and kept out of unwanted trouble.

____Pretty well. I tried to use what I have learned.

____Not so well. I got in more trouble than I wanted.

BEHAVIOR A-B-C'S FOR AN ANGER CUE

A—Something Happens

↓

Anger Cue—heartbeat, muscle tension, etc.

B—What I Choose to Do

↓

Control anger before acting

C—What are the Consequences?

COMMON THOUGHT TRIGGERS

"Awfulizing" Triggers: These are thought triggers that exaggerate the unpleasantness of situations and make them seem worse than they really are.

> *I can't stand the way he does that/says that!*
> *This is the worst thing that could ever happen!*

Demanding Triggers: These are thought triggers that create "demands" out of wants or preferences, as if everyone ought to always do just what we demand that they do, and when they don't, we get angry.

> *He should not say that! He should not do that!*

Overgeneralized Triggers: These are thought triggers that cause us to blow things way out of proportion and that are not really true. These triggers use such words as "always," "never," "everything," and "everybody" to describe what is really much more specific to a given situation.

> *He's always hassling me and never leaves me alone!*
> *Everybody is giving me shit!*

Name-Calling Triggers: These are thought triggers that label a person as something, and they are often unkind, obscene, and designed to increase anger.

> *That son of a bitch (jerk, ass, etc.)!*

REMINDERS

Before:

- Okay, I know it's coming. I can handle it if I stay cool.
- This could be tough, but I can deal with it.
- Just roll with it.
- Take a few deep breaths and stay cool.

During:

- Chill. I can handle this.
- Easy . . . Easy . . . Stay in control.
- Deep breaths . . . Be cool.
- Go slow.

After (*successful* anger control):

- I did pretty good!.
- I'm proud of myself.
- I feel a lot more in control.

After (*unsuccessful* anger control):

- Okay, a setback, but I can handle it.
- What do I need to work on most?.
- It's not the end of the world. At least I'm trying.

STOP AND THINK

What Is The Problem?

- What do I want and what are the obstacles?

What can I do?

- Think about all possible solutions.

What will happen if?

- Think about the worst and the most likely consequences.

Which Should I Choose?

- Which is best for me?

Now Do It!

- What do I need to carry out this solution?

How Did I Do?

- Self-evaluate: Did it work? If not, why?

FINDING ALTERNATIVE SOLUTIONS

When you have plenty of time:

1. Talk to others in order to obtain information or do an Internet search.

2. Brainstorm ideas with friends.

3. Write ideas down on paper.

When you have little time:

4. Recall things that you have done before that required similar skills.

5. Divide a big problem into smaller, more manageable problems.

PROBLEM-SOLVING WORK SHEET

Stop and think:

What is the problem?
- What do I want and what are the obstacles?

What can I do?
- Write down all possible solutions.

What will happen if?
- Write down the worst and most likely consequences for each

Which should I choose?
- Decide which solution is in your best interest.

Now do it!
- Decide if you know how to do this solution on your own.
- Decide what help you need from others to be successful.

References

◆

Achenbach, T. M. (1991. *Manual for the Child Behavior Checklist/4–18 and 1991 profile.* Burlington, VT: University of Vermont Department of Psychiatry.

Adams, D. (1992). Biology does not make men more aggressive than women. In K. Bjorkqvist & P. Niemela (Eds.), *Of mice and women: Aspects of female aggression* (pp. 17–26). Sam Diego, CA: Academic Press.

American Association of University Women. (2001). *Hostile hallways: Bullying, teasing, and sexual harassment in school.* Retrieved June 24, 2003, from *www.aauw.org/research/ girls_education/hostile.cfm.*

Arlington Independent School District. (2003). Retrieved August 28, 2003 from *arlington. k12.tx.us/pdf/coc.pdf.*

Bandmaster, R. F., Smart, L., & Boden, J. M. (1996). Relation of threatened egotism to violence and aggression: The dark side of high self-esteem. *Psychological Review, 103,* 90–113.

Beck, A. T., Rush, A. J., Shaw, B. F., & Emery, G. (1979). *Cognitive therapy of depression.* New York: Guilford Press.

Berkowitz, L. (1993). *Aggression: Its causes, consequences, and control.* New York: McGraw-Hill.

Bosworth, K., Espelage, D. L., & Simon, T. R. (1999.). Factors associated with bullying behavior in middle school students. *Journal of Early Adolescence, 19,* 341–362.

Brener, N. D., Simon, T. R., Krug, E. G., & Lowry, R. (1999). Recent trends in violence-related behaviors among high school students in the United States. *Journal of the American Medical Association, 282,* 440–446.

Brooks, K., Schiraldi, V., & Ziedenberg, J. (2000). *School house hype: Two years later.* Washington, DC: Justice Policy Institute and the Children's Law Center.

Carr, E. G., Horner, R. H., Turnbull, A. P., Marquis, J. G., Magito McLaughlin, D., McAtee, M. L., et al. (1999). *Positive behavior support for people with developmental disabilities:*

A research synthesis (American Association on Mental Retardation Monograph Series). Washington, DC: American Association on Mental Retardation.

Centers for Disease Control and Prevention. (2003). *Youth 2001 online*. Retrieved July 31, 2003 from *www.cdc.gov/nccdphp/dash/yrbs/2001/youth01online.htm*.

Colvin, G., Kameenui, E., & Sugai, G. (1993). Reconceptualizing behavior management and school-wide discipline in general education. *Education and Treatment of Children, 16*, 361–381.

Costenbader, V. K., & Markson, S. (1994). School suspension: A survey of current policies and practices. *NASSP Bulletin, 78*, 103–107.

Covey, S. R. (1992). *Principle-centered leadership*. New York: Simon & Schuster.

Crick, N. R. (1996). The role of overt aggression, relational aggression, and prosocial behavior in the prediction of children's future social adjustment. *Child Development, 67*, 2317–2327.

Crick, N. R. (1997). Engagement in gender normative versus non-normative forms of aggression: Links to social-psychological adjustment. *Developmental Psychology, 33*, 610–617.

Crick, N. R., & Bigbee, M. A. (1998). Relational and overt forms of peer victimization: A multi-informant approach. *Journal of Consulting and Clinical Psychology, 66*, 337–347.

Crick, N. R., & Dodge, K. A. (1994). A review and reformulation of social information-processing mechanisms in children's social adjustment. *Psychological Bulletin, 115*, 74–101.

Crick, N. R., & Grotpeter, J. K. (1995). Relational aggression, gender, and social-psychological adjustment. *Child Development, 66*, 710–722.

Crick, N. R., Nelson, D. A., Morales, J. R., Cullerton-Sen, C., Casas, J. F., & Hickman, S. (2001). Relational victimization in childhood and adolescence: I hurt you through the grapevine. In J. Juvonen & S. Graham (Eds.), *Peer harassment in school: The plight of the vulnerable and victimized* (pp. 196–214). New York: Guilford Press.

Crick, N. R., & Werner, N. E. (1998). Response decision processes in relational and overt aggression. *Child Development, 69*, 1630–1639

Dannemiller, J. L. (Ed.). (2003). Violent children [Special issue]. *Developmental Psychology, 39*(2).

Day, D. M., Golench, C. A., MacDougall, J., & Beals-Gonzalez, C. A. (1995). *School-based violence prevention in Canada: Results of a national survey of policies*. Retrieved August 23, 2003 from *www.sgc.gc.ca/publications/corrections/199502_e.asp*.

Deffenbacher, J. L. (1999). Cognitive-behavioral conceptualization and treatment of anger. *In Session: Psychotherapy in Practice, 55*, 295–309.

DeVoe, J. F., Peter, K., Kaufman, P., Ruddy, S. A., Miller, A. K., Planty, M., et al. (2002). *Indicators of school crime and safety: 2002* (NCES 2003–009/NCJ196753). Washington, DC: U.S. Departments of Education and Justice.

Disney fun facts. (n.d.). Retrieved June 16, 2003, from *hiddenmickeys.org/Secrets.html*.

Dodge, K., & Tomlin, A. (1987). Utilization of self-schemas as a mechanism of interpretational bias in aggressive children. *Social Cognition, 5*, 280–300.

Dodge, K. A. (1991). The structure and function of reactive and proactive aggression. In D. J. Pepler & K. H. Rubin (Eds.), *Development and treatment of childhood aggression* (pp. 201–217). Hillsdale, NJ: Erlbaum.

Dodge, K. A., & Newman, J. P. (1981). Biased decision-making processes in aggressive boys. *Journal of Abnormal Psychology, 90,* 375–379.

Dodge, K. A., Pettit, G. S., McClaskey, C. L., & Brown, M. M. (1986). Social competence in children. *Monographs of the Society for Research in Child Development, 51*(2, Serial No. 213).

Dodge, K. A., Price, J., Bachorowski, J., & Newman, J. (1990). Hostile attributional biases in severely aggressive adolescents. *Journal of Abnormal Psychology, 99,* 385–392.

Doren, B., Bullis, M., & Benz, M. R. (1996). Predictors of victimization experiences of adolescents with disabilities in transition. *Exceptional Children, 63,* 7–18.

Dropout rates in the United States, 1996. (n.d.). Retrieved January 14, 2003, from *nces.ed.gov/pubs98/dropout/98250–06.html.*

D'Zurilla, T. J., & Nezu, A. M. (2001). *Problem-solving therapy: A social competence approach to clinical intervention* (2nd ed.). New York: Springer.

Eber, L., Sugai, G., Smith, C., & Scott, T. M. (2002). Wraparound and positive behavioral interventions and supports in the schools. *Journal of Emotional and Behavioral Disorders, 10,* 136–173.

Eron, L. D., & Slaby, R. G. (1994). Introduction. In L. D. Eron, J. H. Gentry, & P. Schlegel (Eds.), *Reason to hope: A psychological perspective on violence and youth* (pp. 1–22). Washington, DC: American Psychological Association.

Feindler, E. L. (1995). Ideal treatment package for children and adolescents with anger disorders. In H. Kassinove (Ed.), *Anger disorders: Definition, diagnosis, and treatment* (pp. 173–195). Washington, DC: Taylor & Francis.

Feindler, E. L., & Baker, K. (2001). *Current issues in anger management interventions with youth.* Unpublished monograph. (Available from the Department of Psychology, Long Island University/C. W. Post Campus, 720 Northern Boulevard, Brookville, NY 11548-1300)

Feindler, E. L., & Ecton, R. B. (1986). *Adolescent anger control: Cognitive-behavioral techniques.* New York: Allyn & Bacon.

Feindler, E. L., Ecton, R. B., Kingsley, D., & Dubey, D. (1986). Group anger control training for institutionalized psychiatric male adolescents. *Behavior Therapy, 17,* 109–123.

Feindler, E. L., Marriott, S. A., & Iwata, M. (1984). Group anger control training for junior high school delinquents. *Cognitive Therapy and Research, 8,* 299–311.

Feindler, E. L., & Scalley, M. (1998). Anger management groups for violence reduction. In K. C. Stoiber & T. R. Kratochwill (Eds.), *Handbook of group interventions for children and families* (pp. 100–119). Boston: Allyn & Bacon.

Furlong, M., Morrison, G. M., Austin, G., Huh-Kim, J., & Skager, R. (2001). Using student risk factors in school violence surveillance reports: Illustrative examples for enhanced policy formation, implementation, and evaluation. *Law and Policy, 23,* 271–296.

Furlong, M. J., & Smith, D. C. (1994). Assessment of youth's anger, hostility, and aggression using self-report and rating scales. In M. J. Furlong & D. C. Smith (Eds.), *Anger, hostility, and aggression: Assessment, prevention, and intervention strategies for youth* (pp. 167–244). New York: Wiley.

Gallup Organization. (2001, March). *Majority of parents think a school shooting could occur in their community.* Retrieved July 30, 2003, from *www.gallup.com/subscription/?m=f&c_id=9845.*

Garmston, R. J., & Wellman, B. M. (1999). *The adaptive school: A sourcebook for developing collaborative groups.* Norwood, MA: Christopher-Gordon.

Goldstein, A. P., Glick, B., & Gibb, J. C. (1998). *Aggression Replacement Training: A comprehensive intervention for aggressive youth.* Champaign, IL: Research Press.

Goldstein, A. P., Glick, B., Reiner, S., Zimmerman, D., & Coultry, T. (1986). *Aggression replacement training.* Champaign, IL: Research Press.

Goldstein, A. P., & McGinnis, E. (2000). *Skillstreaming the adolescent: New strategies and perspectives for teaching prosocial skills.* Champaign, IL: Research Press.

Gottfredson, D. C. (1997). School-based crime prevention. In L. Sherman, D. Gottfredson, D. Mackenzie, J. Eck, P. Reuter, & S. Bushway (Eds.). *Preventing crime: What works, what doesn't and what's promising.* College Park, MD: Department of Criminology and Criminal Justice.

Greene, J. P., Buka, S. L., Gortmaker, S. L., DeJong, W., & Winsten, J. A. (1997). *Youth violence: The Harvard-MetLife survey of junior and senior high school students.* Retrieved July 23, 2003 from *www.hsph.harvard.edu/press/releases/101498report.html*

Hall, G. E., & Hord, S. M. (1987). *Change in schools: Facilitating the process.* Albany: State University of New York Press.

Hawkins, J. D., Catalano, R. F., Morrison, D. E., O'Donnell, J., Abbott, R. D., & Day, L. E. (1992). The Seattle Social Development Project: Effects of the first four years on protective factors and problem behaviors. In J. McCord & R. Tremblay (Eds.), *The prevention of antisocial behavior in children* (pp. 139–161). New York: Guilford Press.

Herszenhorn, D. M. (2003, May 20). Assaults on teachers are increasing, union says. *The New York Times*, p. 9.

Horner, R., Sugai, G., Lewis-Palmer, T., & Todd, A. (2001). Teaching school-wide behavioral expectations. *Emotional and Behavioral Disorders in Youth, 1,* 77–79, 93–96.

Hudley, C. (1994). Perceptions of intentionality, feelings of anger, and reactive aggression. In M. Furlong & D. Smith, (Eds.), *Anger, hostility, and aggression: Assessment, prevention, and intervention strategies for youth* (pp. 39–56). New York: Wiley.

Hudley, C., Britsch, B., Wakefield, W. D., Smith, T., Demorat, M., & Cho, S. (1998). An attribution retraining program to reduce aggression in elementary school students. *Psychology in the Schools, 35,* 271–282.

Hudley, C. A. (1992). *The reduction of peer directed aggression among highly aggressive African-American boys.* Los Angeles: University of California. (ERIC Document Reproduction Service No. ED346204)

Huesmann, L. R., & Moise, J. (1998). The stability and continuity of aggression from early childhood to young adulthood. In D. J. Flannery & C. R. Huff (Eds.), *Youth violence: Prevention, intervention, and social policy* (pp. 73–95). Washington, DC: American Psychiatric Press.

Hyman, I. A. (1997). *School discipline and school violence: The teacher variance approach.* Boston: Allyn & Bacon.

Jacob, S., & Hartshorne, T. (2003). *Ethics and law for school psychologists* (4th ed.). New York: Wiley.

Johnson, N. G., Roberts, M. C., & Worell, J. (Eds.). (1999). *Beyond appearance: A new look at adolescent girls.* Washington, DC: American Psychological Association.

Kassinove, H., & Sukhodolsky, D. G. (1995). Anger disorders: Basic science and practice issues. In H. Kassinove (Ed.), *Anger disorders: Definition, diagnosis, and treatment* (pp. 2–26). Washington, DC: Taylor & Francis.

Kazdin, A. E. (2001). *Behavior modification in applied settings* (6th ed.). Belmont, CA: Wadsworth/Thomson Learning.

Kendall, P. C., Ronan, K. R., & Epps, J. (1991). Aggression in children/adolescents: Cognitive-behavioral treatment perspectives. In D. J. Pepler & K. H. Rubin (Eds.), *Development and treatment of childhood aggression* (pp. 341–359). Hillsdale, NJ: Erlbaum.

Knoff, H. M. (2002). Best practices in facilitating school reform, organizational change, and strategic planning. In A. Thomas & J. Grimes (Eds.), *Best practices in school psychology* (Vol. 4, pp. 235–244). Silver Spring, MD: National Association of School Psychologists.

Larson, J., & McBride, J. A. (1992). *Think first: Anger and aggression management for secondary level students* (Treatment manual). Whitewater, WI: Author.

Larson, J. (1994). Cognitive-behavioral treatment of anger-induced aggression in the school setting. In M. J. Furlong & D. C. Smith (Eds.), *Anger, hostility, and aggression: Assessment, prevention, and intervention strategies for youth* (pp. 393–440). Brandon, VT: Clinical Psychology Publishing.

Larson, J., & Lochman, J. E. (2002). *Helping schoolchildren cope with anger: A cognitive-behavioral intervention*. New York: Guilford Press.

Larson, J. D. (1991). The effects of a cognitive-behavioral anger-control intervention on the behavior of at-risk middle school students. *Dissertation Abstracts International, 52*(1A), 0117. (UMI No. 9107785)

Larson, J. D. (1992). Anger and aggression management techniques through the Think First curriculum. *Journal of Offender Rehabilitation, 18*(1/2), 101–117.

Larson, J. D., Smith, D. C., & Furlong, M. J. (2002). Best practices in school violence prevention. In A. Thomas & J. Grimes (Eds.), *Best practices in school psychology* (Vol. 4, pp. 1081–1098). Silver Spring, MD: National Association of School Psychologists.

Leschied, A., Cummings, A., Van Brunschot, M., Cunningham, A., & Saunders, A. (2000). *Female adolescent aggression: A review of the literature and the correlates of aggression* (User Report No. 2000–04). Ottawa, CA: Solicitor General Canada.

Lipsey, M., & Derzon, J. (1998). Predictors of violent or serious delinquency in adolescence and early adulthood: A synthesis on longitudinal research. In R. Loeber & D. Farrington (Eds.), *Serious and violent juvenile offenders: Risk factors and successful interventions* (pp. 86–105). Thousand Oaks, CA: Sage.

Lochman, J. E., & Curry, J. F. (1986). Effects of social problem-solving training and self-instruction training with aggressive boys. *Journal of Consulting and Clinical Psychology, 63*, 549–559.

Lochman, J. E., & Dodge, K. A. (1994). Social-cognitive processes of severely violent, moderately aggressive, and nonaggressive boys. *Journal of Consulting and Clinical Psychology,62*, 366–374.

Lochman, J. E., Dunn, S. E., & Wagner, E. E. (1997). Anger. In G. Bear, K. Minke, & A. Thomas (Eds.), *Children's needs II* (pp. 149–160). Silver Spring, MD: National Association of School Psychologists.

Lochman, J. E., & Lampron, L. B. (1986). Situational social problem-solving skills and self-esteem of aggressive and nonaggressive boys. *Journal of Abnormal Child Psychology 14*, 605–617.

Lochman, J. E., Meyer, B. L., Rabiner, D. L., & White, K. J. (1991). Parameters influencing social problem-solving of aggressive children. In R. Prinz (Ed.), *Advances in behavioral assessment of child and families* (Vol. 5, pp. 31–63). Greenwich, CT: JAI Press.

Lochman, J. E., Whidby, J. M., & FitzGerald, D. P. (2000). In P. C. Kendall (Ed.), *Child and adolescent therapy* (2nd ed., pp. 31–87). New York: Guilford Press.

Lochman, J. E., White, K. J., & Wayland, K. K. (1991). Cognitive-behavioral assessment and treatment with aggressive children. In P. C. Kendall (Ed.), *Child and adolescent therapy: Cognitive-behavioral procedures* (pp. 25–65). New York: Guilford Press.

Lockwood, D. (1997). *Violence among high school and middle school students: Analysis and implication for prevention.* (NCJ Publication No. 166363). Washington, DC: U.S. Department of Justice.

Loeber, R. (1988). The natural history of juvenile conduct problems, delinquency, and associated substance use: Evidence for developmental progressions. In B. B. Lahey & A. E. Kazdin (Eds.), *Advances in clinical child psychology* (Vol. 11, pp. 73–124). New York: Plenum.

Loeber, R. (1990). Development and risk factors of juvenile antisocial behavior and delinquency. *Clinical Psychology Review, 10,* 1–41.

Madison Metropolitan School District. (2003). Retrieved August 1, 2003 from *www.madison.k12.wi.us/policies/4502.htm.*

Massey, O. T., Armstrong, K. H., & Boroughs, M. (2003). *The Think First anger management curriculum: Effectiveness for secondary students under two conditions of implementation.* Tampa, FL: University of South Florida, Louis de la Parte Florida Mental Health Institute.

Matsumoto, D. (2001a). Culture and emotion. In D. Matsumoto (Ed.), *The handbook of culture and psychology* (pp. 171–194). New York: Oxford University Press.

Matsumoto, D. (2001b). Cross-cultural psychology in the 21st century. In J. S. Halonen & S. F. Davis (Eds.), *The many faces of psychological research in the 21st century.* Society for the Teaching of Psychology. Available online at *teachpsych.lemoyne.edu/teachpsych/faces/facesindex.html.*

Meichenbaum, D. (1985). *Stress inoculation training: A practitioner's guidebook.* New York: Allyn & Bacon.

Meichenbaum, D. (2001). *Treatment of individuals with anger control problems and aggressive behaviors: A clinical handbook.* Clearwater, FL: Institute Press.

Meichenbaum, D. H., & Goodman, J. (1971). Training impulsive children to talk to themselves. *Journal of Abnormal Psychology, 77,* 115–126.

Milwaukee Catalyst. (2001). *Beyond suspensions: Safe and orderly schools that educate all students.* Milwaukee, WI: Author.

Moffitt, T. E. (1993). Adolescence-limited and life-course persistent antisocial behavior: A developmental taxonomy. *Psychological Review, 100,* 674–701.

Morgan-D'Atrio, C., Northrup, J., LaFleur, L., & Spera, S. (1996). Toward prescriptive alternatives to suspensions: A preliminary evaluation. *Behavioral Disorders, 21,* 190–200.

Nansel, T. R., Overpeck, M., Pilla, R. S., Ruan, W. J., Simons-Morton, B., & Scheidt, P. (2001). Bullying behaviors among U.S. youth: Prevalence and association with psychosocial adjustment. *Journal of the American Medical Association, 285*(16), 2094–2100.

Nanus, B. (1992). *Visionary leadership: Creating a compelling sense of direction for your organization*. San Francisco: Jossey-Bass.

Nasby, W., Hayden, B., & DePaulo, B. M. (1979). Attributional biases among aggressive boys to interpret unambiguous social stimuli as displays of hostility. *Journal of Abnormal Psychology, 89,* 459–468.

National Association of School Psychologists. (2002). Position statement on school violence. Retrieved July 27, 2003 from *http://www.nasponline.org/information/pospaper_violence.html*.

National Center for Educational Statistics. (2001). Enrollment trends, public & private schools. Retrieved July 18, 2003 from *http://nces.ed.gov/fastfacts/display.asp?id=65*

National Center for Educational Statistics. (2003). The condition of education 2003. Retrieved June 19, 2003, from *nces.ed.gov/pubsearch/pubsinfo.asp?pubid=2003067*.

National Criminal Justice Reference Service. (n.d.). *Overview of the truancy problem.* Retrieved December 16, 2003, from *www.ncjrs.org/html/ojjdp/jjbul2001_9_1/page1.html*.

National Research Council. (1993). *Understanding and preventing violence.* Washington, DC: National Academy Press.

National School Safety Center. (2003). *School-associated violent deaths report.* Retrieved June 23, 2003, from *www.nssc1.org/*.

Nelson, W. M., & Finch, A. J. (2000). *Children's Inventory of Anger (CHIA): Manual.* Los Angeles, CA: Western Psychological Service.

Nickerson, K. F. (2003). *Anger in adolescents: The effectiveness of a brief cognitive-behavioral anger management training program for reducing attitudinal and behavioral expressions of anger.* Unpublished doctoral dissertation, Cappella University, Minneapolis, MN.

Novaco, R. W. (1975). *Anger control: The development and treatment of an experimental treatment.* Lexington, MA: Heath.

Novaco, R. W. (1985). Anger and its therapeutic regulation. In M. A. Chesney & R. H. Rosenman (Eds.), *Anger and hostility in cardiovascular and behavioral disorders* (pp. 203–226). New York: Hemisphere.

Oakley, E., & Krug, D. (1991). *Enlightened leadership: Getting to the heart of change.* New York: Simon & Schuster.

O'Donnell, C. R. (2001). Trends, risk factors, prevention, and recommendations. *Law and Policy, 23,* 409–416.

Office of Special Education Programs. (2001). *Twenty-third annual report to congress on the implementation of the Individuals with Disabilities in Education Act.* Retrieved January 30, 2003, from *www.ed.gov/offices/OSERS/OSEP/Products/OSEP2001AnlRpt/index.html*.

Olweus, D. (1979). Stability of aggressive reaction patterns in males: A review. *Psychological Bulletin, 86,* 852–875.

Olweus, D. (1991). Bully/victim problems among school children: Basic facts and effects of a school based intervention program. In D. J. Pepler & K. H. Rubin (Eds.), *The development and treatment of childhood aggression* (pp. 411–448). Hillsdale, NJ: Erlbaum.

O'Neill, R. E., Horner, R. H., Albin, R. W., Sprague, J. R., Storey, K., & Newton, J. S.

(1997). *Functional assessment and program development for problem behavior: A practical handbook* (2nd ed.). Pacific Grove, CA: Brooks/Cole.

Patterson, G. R., DeBaryshe, B. D., & Ramsey, E. (1989). A developmental perspective on antisocial behavior. *American Psychologist, 44*, 329–335.

Patterson, G. R., Reid, J. B., & Dishion, T. J. (1992). *Antisocial boys*. Eugene, OR: Castalia.

Pepler, D. J., & Craig, W. (1999). *Aggressive girls: Development of disorder and outcomes* (Research Report No. 57). Toronto, Ontario, Canada: York University, LeMarsh Center for Research on Violence and Conflict Resolution.

Pepler, D. J., Craig, W. M., & Roberts, W. I. (1998). Observations of aggressive and nonaggressive children on the school playground. *Merrill–Palmer Quarterly, 44*(1), 55–76.

Pepler, D. J., King, G., & Byrd, W. (1991). A social-cognitively based social skills training program for aggressive children. In D. J. Pepler & K. H. Rubin (Eds.), *Development and treatment of childhood aggression* (pp. 361–379). Hillsdale, NJ: Erlbaum.

Pepler, D. J., Madsen, K. C., Webster, C. D., & Levine, K. S. (Eds.). (2004). *The development and treatment of girlhood aggression*. Mahwah, NJ: Erlbaum.

Pepler, D. J., & Sedighdeilami, F. (1998, October). *Aggressive girls in Canada* (Report No. W-98–30E). Applied Research Branch, Strategic Policy, Retrieved June 1, 2001, from the Human Resources Development Canada, Hull, Quebec, Canada. Human Resources Development Canada Web site: *www.hrdc-drhc.gc.ca/stratpol/arb/publications/research/abw-98-30e.shtml.*

Peterson, R. L., Larson, J., & Skiba, R. (2001). School violence prevention: Current status and policy recommendations. *Law and Policy, 23*, 245–372.

Pettit, G. S. (1997). Aggression. In G. C. Bear, K. M. Minke, & A. Thomas (Eds.), *Children's needs: II. Development, problems, and alternatives* (pp. 135–137). Bethesda, MD: National Association of School Psychologists.

Redding, R. E., & Shalf, S. M. (2001). The legal context of school violence: The effectiveness of federal, state, and local law enforcement efforts to reduce gun violence. *Law & Policy, 23*, 297–344.

Reynolds, C. R., & Kamphaus, R. W. (1992). *Behavior Assessment System for Children (BASC)*. Circle Pines, MN: American Guidance Services.

Rokke, P. D., & Rehm, L. P. (2001). Self-management strategies. In K. S. Dobson (Ed.), *Handbook of cognitive-behavioral therapies* (pp. 173–210). New York: Guilford Press.

Rose, L. C., & Gallup, A. C. (2003). *The thirty-third annual Phi Delta Kappa/Gallup poll of the public's attitude toward the public schools*. Retrieved July 29, 2003, from *www.pdkintl.org/kappan/k0109gal.htm#3a.*

Rotter, J. (1966). Generalized expectancies for internal versus external control of reinforcements. *Psychological Monographs, 80*, Whole No. 609.

Sattler, J. (1997). *Clinical and forensic interviewing of children and families: Guidelines for the mental health, education, pediatric, and child maltreatment fields*. La Mesa, CA: Sattler.

Sattler, J. (2002). *Assessment of children: Behavioral and clinical applications* (4th ed.). La Mesa, CA: Sattler.

Senge, P., Cambron-McCabe, N. H., Lucas, T., Kleiner, A., Dutton, J., & Smith, B. (2000).

Schools that learn: A fifth discipline fieldbook for educators, parents and everyone who cares about education. New York: Doubleday.

Shannon, M. M., & McCall, D. S. (2003). *Zero tolerance policies on context: A preliminary investigation to identify actions to improve school discipline and school safety.* Retrieved 9-1-03 from *www.safehealthyschools.org/whatsnew/capzerotolerance.htm*

Skiba, R. J. (2000). *Zero tolerance, zero evidence: An analysis of school disciplinary practice* (Policy Research Report #SRS2). University of Indiana, Indiana Education Policy Center.

Skiba, R., & Peterson, R. (1999, January). The dark side of zero tolerance: Can punishment lead to safe schools? *Phi Delta Kappan, 372–382.*

Slaby, R. G., & Guerra, N. G. (1988). Cognitive mediators of aggression in adolescent offenders: 1. Assessment. *Developmental Psychology, 24, 580–588.*

Smith, D. C., Furlong, M., Bates, M., & Laughlin, J. D. (1998). The development of the multi-dimensional school anger inventory for males. *Psychology in the Schools, 35, 1–15.*

Smith, D. C., Larson, J. D., DeBaryshe, B. D., & Salzman, M. (2000). Anger management for youth: What works and for whom? In D. S. Sandhu (Ed.), *Violence in American schools: A practical guide for counselors.* Reston, VA: American Counseling Association.

Spielberger, C. D. (1999). *The State–Trait Anger Expression Inventory–2 Manual.* Lutz, FL: Psychological Assessment Resources.

Spielberger, C. D., Reheiser, E. C., & Sydeman, S. J. (1999). Measuring the experience, expression, and control of anger. In H. Kassinove (Ed.), *Anger disorders: Definition, diagnosis, and treatment* (pp. 49–65). Washington, DC: Taylor & Francis.

Sprick, R. (Speaker). (1998). *Behavioral interventions for at-risk students* (Cassette Recording WS17a). Silver Spring, MD: National Association of School Psychologists.

Sprick, R. S., Borgmeier, C., & Nolet, V. (2002). Prevention and management of behavior problems in the secondary schools. In M. A. Shinn, H. M. Walker, & G. Stoner (Eds.), *Interventions for academic and behavior problems: II. Preventive and remedial approaches* (pp. 373–403). Bethesda, MD: National Association of School Psychologists.

Stein, R. P., Richin, R. A., Banyon, R., Banyon, F., & Stein, M. F. (2000). *Connecting character to content: Helping students do the right thing.* Alexandria, VA: Association for Curriculum Development.

Striepling, S. H. (1997). The low aggression classroom: A teacher's view. In A. P. Goldstein & J. C. Conoley (Eds.), *School violence intervention: A practical handbook* (pp. 23–45). New York: Guilford Press.

Sugai, G., & Horner, R. (1999). Discipline and behavioral support: Preferred processes and practices. *Effective School Practices, 17, 10–22.*

Sugai, G., Horner, R. H., Dunlap, G., Hieneman, M., Lewis, T., Nelson, C. M., et al. (1999). *Applying positive behavioral support and functional behavioral assessment in schools* (Technical Assistance Guide 1 Version 1.4.4, 12/01/99). Washington, DC: OSEP Center on Positive Behavioral Interventions and Support.

Sugai, G., Horner, R., & Gresham, F. (2002). Behaviorally effective school environments. In M. A. Shinn, H. M. Walker, & G. Stoner (Eds.), *Interventions for academic and behavior problems: II. Preventive and remedial approaches* (pp. 315–350). Bethesda, MD: National Association of School Psychologists.

Sugai, G., & Lewis, T. J. (Eds.). (1999). *Providing positive behavioral support for children with challenging behaviors.* Arlington, VA: Council for Exceptional Children.

Sugai, G., Sprague, J. R., Horner, R. H., & Walker, H. M. (2001). Preventing school violence: The use of office discipline referrals to assess and monitor school-wide discipline interventions. In H. H. Walker & M. H. Epstein (Eds.), *Making schools safer and violence free: Critical issues, solutions, and recommended practices* (pp. 50–57). Austin, TX: Pro-Ed.

Tolan, P., & Guerra, N. (1994). *What works in reducing adolescent violence: An empirical review of the field.* (Center Paper No. 001). Boulder, CO: Center for the Study and Prevention of Violence, Institute for Behavioral Sciences, University of Colorado.

Tolan, P. H., Guerra, N. G., & Kendall, P. C. (1995). A developmental-ecological perspective on antisocial behavior in children and adolescents: Toward a unified risk and intervention framework. *Journal of Consulting and Clinical Psychology, 63,* 579–584.

Underwood, M. (Ed.). (2003). *Social aggression among girls.* New York: Guilford Press.

U.S. Department of Education. (1998). *Early warning, timely response: A guide to safe schools.* Washington, DC: Author.

Vossekuil, B., Fine, R., Reddy, M., Borum, R., & Modzeleski, W. (2002).*The final report and findings of the Safe School Initiative: Implications for the prevention of school attacks in the United States.* Retrieved June 23, 2003, from *www.secretservice.gov/ntac/ssi_final_report.pdf.*

Walker, H. (1993). Antisocial behavior in school. *Journal of Emotional and Behavior Disorders, 1,* 20–24.

Walker, H. M., Colvin, G., & Ramsey, E. (1995). *Antisocial behavior in schools: Strategies and best practices.* Pacific Grove, CA: Brooks/Cole.

Walker, H. M., Homer, R. H., Sugai, G., Bullis, M., Sprague, J. R., Bricker, D., & Kaufman, M. J. (1996). Integrated approaches to preventing antisocial behavior patterns among school-age children and youth. *Journal of Emotional and Behavioral Disorders, 4,* 194–209.

Walinsky, A. (1995, July). The crisis of public order. *The Atlantic Monthly,* 39–54.

Walker, H. M., Ramsey, E., & Gresham, F. M. (2004). *Antisocial behavior in school* (2nd ed.). Belmont, CA: Wadsworth/Thomson Learning.

Walsh, M. M., Pepler, D. J., & Levene, K. S. (2002). A model intervention for girls with disruptive behaviour problems: The Earlscourt Girls Connection. Canadian *Journal of Counselling, 36,* 297–310.

Watson, T. S., & Steege, M. W. (2003). *Conducting school-based functional behavioral assessments: A practitioner's guide.* New York: Guilford Press.

Wisconsin State Statutes, 120.13(1)(a) (2003).

Index

◆